The DMSO Master Guide

A Complete Healing Guide to Dimethyl Sulfoxide with Over 100 Remedies for Pain, Detox, Chronic Conditions, and More

Elena Walker

Copyright Page

Title: The DMSO Master Guide: A Complete Healing Guide to Dimethyl Sulfoxide with Over 100 Remedies for Pain, Detox, Chronic Conditions, and More

Author: Elena Walker

Copyright © 2025 by Elena Walker.

All rights reserved. No part of this book may be reproduced, distributed, or transmitted in any form or by any means, including photocopying, recording, or other electronic or mechanical methods, without prior written permission from the author, except in the case of brief quotations embodied in reviews and certain other non-commercial uses permitted by copyright law. For permission requests, please contact the author at the address below.

Disclaimer
The information contained in this book is for educational and informational purposes only and is not intended as medical advice. The use of DMSO should always be undertaken with caution and under the supervision of a qualified healthcare professional. The author is not responsible for any adverse effects, consequences, or outcomes resulting from the application or misapplication of the information presented in this book.

This book does not substitute for professional medical diagnosis, advice, or treatment. The author makes no representations or warranties with respect to the accuracy, applicability, or completeness of the content. Readers should consult their healthcare provider or other qualified medical professionals regarding any questions or concerns they may have about their health, medications, or treatment plans.

This book also discusses some off-label uses of DMSO. The inclusion of such uses is for informational purposes only and does not constitute endorsement or recommendation. Always consult with a healthcare professional before using any substance or implementing any treatment.

The author assumes no liability for inaccuracies or omissions in the content or for damages of any kind arising from the use of this book or the materials contained herein.

DMSO products and related recommendations mentioned in this book may be subject to regulations that vary by region or country. It is the responsibility of the reader to ensure compliance with local laws and regulations before use.

First Edition: January 2025

TABLE OF CONTENTS

Preface 1

Introduction 5

Part I: The Science and History of DMSO 13
Chapter 1: Understanding DMSO 14
Chapter 2: The Evolution of DMSO 23

Part II: Safe Use and Preparation 37
Chapter 3: Preparing to Use DMSO 38
Chapter 4: Safety and Precautions 54

Part III: Remedies by Condition 67
Chapter 5: Pain Relief 68
Chapter 6: Skin Health and Wound Healing 85
Chapter 7: Respiratory and Immune Support 99
Chapter 8: Digestive and Detoxification Remedies 115
Chapter 9: Bone and Joint Health 131

Part IV: Advanced Applications 147
Chapter 10: Combining DMSO with Other Therapies 148
Chapter 11: Veterinary and Sports Medicine 164

Part V: Incorporating DMSO into Holistic Health 171

Chapter 12: Integrating DMSO into a Wellness Routine 172

Chapter 13: Synergistic Effects of DMSO 184

Part VI: Advancements and Practical Applications 197

Chapter 14: Innovations and Research 198

Chapter 15: FAQs and Myths Debunked 207

Chapter 16: Quick Reference Guides 212

Conclusion 217

References 220

PREFACE

If you're reading this, chances are you've heard about DMSO. Maybe someone mentioned it as a miracle for chronic pain, a natural anti-inflammatory, or a powerful tool for healing that mainstream medicine often overlooks. Or perhaps you stumbled across it in your own search for answers, intrigued by its reputation yet uncertain about how it works or whether it's worth exploring. Whatever brought you here, welcome. You're in the right place.

When I first encountered DMSO, I was like many of you—curious, skeptical, and maybe even a little overwhelmed. It's not every day that you come across a substance that can penetrate the skin, deliver nutrients, reduce inflammation, and support healing, all in one bottle. But that's exactly what DMSO does. Derived from trees and used for decades in medical and industrial applications, this unassuming compound is a natural powerhouse. Yet, despite its incredible potential, it remains one of the best-kept secrets in holistic health.

Let me be clear: I'm not a scientist or a doctor by trade. My expertise didn't come from a lab or a classroom; it came from necessity. Years ago, I was frustrated with conventional treatments that addressed symptoms but not the root cause. I needed something more—a tool that could help me regain control over my health. That's when DMSO entered my life.

At first, I approached it with caution. The more I read about its benefits, the more questions I had. How could something so versatile not be widely known or recommended? Why was it celebrated by some and dismissed by others? What was the science behind its effects, and how could I use it safely? Armed with curiosity and a healthy dose of skepticism, I began my journey into the world of DMSO.

What I discovered was transformative. Through research, personal experimentation, and guidance from experts in the field, I learned how to harness the power of DMSO for myself and my family. Chronic pain became manageable. Scars I thought were permanent began to fade. Friends and loved ones who tried it found relief from conditions they'd been struggling with for years. It wasn't magic, and it wasn't instant, but it was real.

Over time, I became the go-to person in my circle for all things DMSO. People would ask, "How do I use it? What dilution is safe? Can it help with this or that?" The questions were endless, and I realized there was a need for a clear, practical guide—a resource that could demystify DMSO and make it accessible to everyone, whether they were experienced in natural remedies or just beginning to explore them. That's how this book came to be.

This isn't just a collection of facts and figures. It's a roadmap, drawn from my own experiences and the stories of countless others who have used DMSO to improve their lives. It's about more than just how to use DMSO— it's about empowering you to take charge of your health, to ask questions, and to make informed choices that align with your needs.

In the chapters ahead, we'll cover everything you need to know about DMSO. We'll start with the basics—what it is, how it works, and why it's so effective. You'll learn about its history, its applications in both mainstream and alternative medicine, and the science behind its unique properties. From there, we'll dive into practical tips for using DMSO safely and effectively, including dilution ratios, application methods, and troubleshooting common issues.

But this book is about more than just the "how." It's about the "why." Why DMSO can be a game-changer for pain relief, skin health, inflammation, and more. Why it's worth considering as part of a holistic approach to wellness. And why, despite its many benefits, it's often misunderstood or underutilized.

I've also included recipes and remedies tailored to specific conditions, from chronic pain and arthritis to skin rejuvenation and detoxification. These aren't just theoretical suggestions—they're tried-and-true methods that I, and many others, have used with success. Whether you're dealing with a persistent health challenge or simply looking to support your body's natural healing processes, you'll find practical, actionable advice in these pages.

Healing is a deeply personal journey, and there's no one-size-fits-all solution. DMSO is an incredible tool, but like any tool, it's most effective when used with care and understanding. That's why I've taken the time to include not just instructions, but context—real-life stories, insights from experts, and the lessons I've learned along the way. My hope is that this book will serve as a trusted companion on your path to better health, offering both knowledge and inspiration.

So, whether you're new to DMSO or looking to deepen your understanding, I invite you to explore these pages with an open mind. Take your time, experiment thoughtfully, and trust your intuition. Healing isn't a straight line, but every step you take brings you closer to balance and vitality. You have the power to transform your health, and I'm honored to share this journey with you.

Let's begin.

INTRODUCTION

1.1 DMSO: The Versatile Healer

DMSO, or dimethyl sulfoxide, is an exceptional compound with a legacy as unique as its properties. Derived from trees during the papermaking process, this simple yet powerful molecule has captivated scientists, doctors, and natural health enthusiasts for decades. What makes DMSO so remarkable isn't just what it does, but how it does it. It's a solvent, a carrier, an anti-inflammatory agent, and a healer—all rolled into one.

To understand why DMSO is often called the "miracle molecule," you need to know a bit about how it works. Unlike most substances, DMSO has the rare ability to penetrate the skin and cellular membranes, delivering its therapeutic properties directly to the body's tissues. But it doesn't stop there—it can also carry other beneficial substances along with it. This dual function makes DMSO a versatile tool for addressing pain, inflammation, and a host of other conditions, from the surface of the skin to the body's deepest tissues.

What sets DMSO apart isn't just its effectiveness, but its range of applications. Used topically, it can reduce swelling and soothe aching joints. When combined with other ingredients, it enhances their delivery and potency. In more advanced medical settings, DMSO has even been explored for its potential in treating serious conditions like interstitial cystitis, traumatic brain injuries, and certain cancers. Its versatility is staggering, yet it remains underappreciated outside niche communities of health-conscious individuals and holistic practitioners.

For me, DMSO represents a bridge between nature and science—a natural compound backed by decades of research and clinical use. It's one of the rare remedies that feels both ancient and cutting-edge, with roots in the natural world and applications in modern medicine. But perhaps what's most compelling about DMSO is its accessibility. Unlike many pharmaceuticals, it doesn't require a prescription, and it's affordable enough to be within reach for most people. It's not a cure-all, but it's a tool that can empower individuals to take control of their health in ways they may never have thought possible.

Despite its impressive benefits, DMSO isn't without its quirks. It has a distinct garlic-like smell, a polarizing reputation in the medical community, and a learning curve when it comes to safe and effective use. These challenges, however, pale in comparison to its potential to support healing and wellness. For those willing to explore it with an open mind and a thoughtful approach, DMSO offers possibilities that are as profound as they are practical.

In the chapters ahead, we'll explore the science behind DMSO, its applications for a variety of health concerns, and how you can integrate it into your wellness routine. Whether you're seeking relief from chronic pain, looking to rejuvenate your skin, or simply curious about this intriguing compound, you'll find answers and inspiration in the pages to come. DMSO is more than a remedy—it's a gateway to empowered, informed healing.

1.2 From Nature to Medicine: A Transformative Journey

The story of DMSO is one of discovery, persistence, and transformation. From its humble beginnings as a byproduct of the wood pulping industry to its evolution as a medical and therapeutic marvel, DMSO has carved a unique path in the world of science and natural health. Its journey reflects not only the ingenuity of researchers but also the resilience of a substance that refused to be ignored.

DMSO was first synthesized in the 19th century by Russian chemist Alexander Zaytsev. At the time, its potential as a solvent was recognized, but it wasn't until the mid-20th century that its remarkable biological properties came to light. Scientists discovered that DMSO could penetrate skin and cellular membranes without damaging them—a capability that set it apart from almost every other compound. This discovery was a breakthrough, offering new possibilities for drug delivery, pain management, and inflammation reduction.

In the 1960s, Dr. Stanley Jacob at the University of Oregon conducted pioneering research into DMSO's medical applications. His studies revealed its potential to reduce inflammation, alleviate pain, and even protect cells from injury. This sparked widespread interest, and DMSO quickly became the focus of both excitement and controversy. On one hand, it showed promise as a versatile treatment for conditions ranging from arthritis to interstitial cystitis. On the other, its rapid rise to prominence left some in the medical community wary, particularly as DMSO's side effects and long-term safety had yet to be fully understood.

Regulatory hurdles soon followed. In the United States, the FDA approved DMSO for specific uses, such as treating interstitial cystitis, but hesitated to endorse it for broader applications. This hesitation, coupled with the compound's distinct garlic-like odor and its ability to carry substances into the bloodstream, slowed its adoption in mainstream medicine. However, it gained a devoted following among natural health practitioners, holistic healers, and individuals who valued its affordability and accessibility.

What's remarkable about DMSO is its ability to bridge the gap between nature and medicine. Derived from trees, it retains its organic roots while offering scientifically validated benefits. It's a testament to the power of natural substances to meet modern medical challenges, providing solutions that are both effective and sustainable. DMSO's journey is also a reminder of the importance of curiosity and open-mindedness in scientific exploration. Without researchers willing to look beyond its industrial origins, DMSO might have remained an obscure solvent, its healing potential untapped.

Today, DMSO occupies a unique space in the world of health and wellness. It's a tool for those seeking alternatives to conventional treatments, a resource for scientists exploring new frontiers, and a lifeline for individuals managing chronic conditions. Its transformative journey from industrial byproduct to therapeutic ally is not just a story of scientific discovery—it's a call to consider the untapped potential of the natural world.

As we continue to explore DMSO in this book, you'll see how its history shapes its applications today. You'll learn about the challenges it faced, the victories it achieved, and the lessons it offers for anyone willing to embrace innovation and self-empowered healing. DMSO's story is still being written, and you're now a part of it.

1.3 Why This Guide Matters: A Practical Approach

The world of health and wellness is vast, and for those seeking alternative or complementary remedies, it can feel overwhelming. DMSO stands out as a beacon of possibility, but for many, it also raises questions. What exactly is it? How do you use it safely? And perhaps most importantly, does it live up to its reputation as a "miracle molecule"? This guide was created to answer those questions and more, serving as both a roadmap and a companion for your journey with DMSO.

There's no shortage of information about DMSO online and in niche communities. Yet, much of it is fragmented, overly technical, or riddled with misinformation. Some sources tout it as a cure-all, while others dismiss it outright due to outdated biases or limited understanding. The truth, as is often the case, lies somewhere in between. DMSO is neither a magic bullet nor a mere placebo. It's a powerful tool—one that requires knowledge, care, and context to be used effectively.

This guide bridges the gap between curiosity and confidence. It's designed for everyone, whether you're entirely new to DMSO or have dabbled with it before but want a deeper understanding. My goal isn't just to explain what DMSO is or how it works—it's to empower you to make informed decisions that align with your health goals.

What sets this book apart is its practical approach. Instead of burying you in technical jargon, I've distilled the essentials into clear, actionable insights. You'll find detailed instructions on how to dilute and apply DMSO, tips for avoiding common mistakes, and recipes tailored to specific conditions.

Whether you're managing chronic pain, looking to rejuvenate your skin, or exploring natural detoxification, there's a chapter here for you.

But beyond the how-to, this guide delves into the "why." Why does DMSO work so effectively for certain conditions? Why has it remained a hidden gem despite decades of research and clinical use? And why should you consider integrating it into your wellness routine? By exploring these questions, my hope is to provide not just answers, but clarity—a framework that helps you see DMSO not as an isolated remedy, but as part of a larger, holistic approach to health.

One of the things I've learned in my own journey with DMSO is the importance of context. Healing isn't just about the substances we use; it's about how we approach them. It's about understanding our bodies, respecting the tools we choose, and being open to experimentation and learning. This guide reflects that philosophy. It's grounded in research, enriched by personal experience, and designed to inspire curiosity and confidence.

For those who may feel hesitant or unsure, let me say this: DMSO isn't as intimidating as it might seem. Yes, it has a distinct smell and a reputation for being unconventional. But with a little guidance, it's incredibly accessible and easy to use. This book breaks down the process step by step, so you can feel confident in your choices and get the most out of your DMSO journey.

I believe in the power of informed self-care. We live in a world where it's easy to hand over responsibility for our health to others—doctors, pharmaceuticals, and institutions. While these have their place, there's also immense value in taking an active role in our own wellness. DMSO is one of those tools that puts power back in your hands. It's affordable, effective, and versatile, and it doesn't require a prescription or a degree in biochemistry to use. What it does require is an open mind, a little patience, and the willingness to explore.

This guide is my way of sharing what I've learned, not as an absolute authority, but as someone who has walked this path before you. It's a practical resource, a collection of insights, and a source of encouragement. My hope is that it will demystify DMSO and help you see it for what it truly is: a remarkable gift from nature, ready to support you in achieving better health.

Part I

THE SCIENCE AND HISTORY OF DMSO

Chapter 1

UNDERSTANDING DMSO

1.1 Origins and Discovery: A Byproduct of Nature

Every remarkable discovery begins somewhere, and the story of DMSO is no exception. While today it's hailed for its versatility and healing potential, its origins are surprisingly humble, rooted in the industrial processes of papermaking. Derived from lignin, a natural polymer found in the cell walls of plants, DMSO emerged as a byproduct during the production of pulp and paper. For decades, it was viewed merely as an industrial solvent, valuable for its ability to dissolve both organic and inorganic compounds. Yet beneath this utilitarian role lay the seeds of something extraordinary.

DMSO, or dimethyl sulfoxide, was first synthesized in 1866 by Russian chemist Alexander Zaytsev. At the time, its chemical properties intrigued scientists, but it remained little more than a laboratory curiosity. It wasn't until the mid-20th century that researchers began to unravel its broader potential. The pivotal moment came when scientists discovered DMSO's unique ability to penetrate skin and cellular membranes without causing damage. This finding was unprecedented, opening the door to applications in medicine, pharmacology, and beyond.

What made DMSO truly extraordinary was its ability to transport other substances through the skin and into the bloodstream. This property—known as transdermal absorption—set it apart from virtually every other compound known at the time. Suddenly, DMSO was no longer just a solvent; it was a potential game-changer for drug delivery, inflammation control, and tissue healing.

In the 1960s, Dr. Stanley Jacob at the University of Oregon became one of the earliest champions of DMSO's medical potential. His research demonstrated its ability to reduce swelling, alleviate pain, and protect cells from injury. Dr. Jacob's work marked the beginning of a new chapter for DMSO, transforming it from an industrial byproduct into a substance with profound therapeutic applications.

Despite its promise, DMSO's journey to mainstream acceptance was anything but smooth. Its rapid rise to prominence sparked both excitement and controversy. The medical community marveled at its potential, yet many remained cautious, wary of its unconventional origins and the lack of long-term safety data at the time. Adding to the skepticism was DMSO's most notorious quirk: its distinct garlic-like odor, a harmless but polarizing side effect caused by the compound's metabolism in the body.

Even in the face of skepticism, DMSO's versatility could not be ignored. Beyond its medicinal applications, it found uses in agriculture, veterinary medicine, and cryopreservation, where its ability to protect cells during freezing made it invaluable for preserving biological samples. This adaptability further cemented its reputation as a substance worth exploring.

Today, DMSO is recognized as a bridge between nature and innovation. Its origins as a simple byproduct remind us of the untapped potential that lies within the natural world, waiting to be discovered. As you continue through this book, you'll see how this unassuming compound evolved into a powerful tool for healing and wellness, proving that sometimes the most extraordinary solutions come from the most unexpected places.

1.2 Chemistry of DMSO: What Makes It Unique

To truly appreciate DMSO and its myriad applications, it's essential to delve into its chemistry—the very foundation that gives this molecule its remarkable properties. Now, I promise not to turn this into a dense chemistry lecture, but understanding what makes DMSO unique will empower you to use it more effectively and safely.

At its core, DMSO stands for **dimethyl sulfoxide**. Its molecular formula is $(CH_3)_2SO$, which means it consists of two methyl groups (CH_3) attached to a sulfur atom that's double-bonded to an oxygen atom. This simple structure belies the complex and versatile nature of the molecule. What sets DMSO apart chemically is its **polar aprotic solvent** status. Let me break that down.

A **polar** molecule has an uneven distribution of electron density, which allows it to interact with other polar substances—think of how water dissolves salt. An **aprotic** solvent, on the other hand, lacks a hydrogen atom connected to an electronegative atom, meaning it doesn't donate hydrogen bonds. This combination is relatively rare and gives DMSO the ability to dissolve both polar and nonpolar compounds. In practical terms, DMSO can mix with water, oils, and a wide range of organic substances, making it an exceptional carrier.

One of the most fascinating aspects of DMSO is its **ability to penetrate biological membranes**. This is due to its small molecular size and polar nature, allowing it to pass through skin, mucous membranes, and even cellular walls without causing damage. This permeability is why DMSO is so effective as a topical agent—it doesn't just sit on the skin's surface; it goes deeper, reaching tissues and cells that other substances can't access as readily.

But DMSO isn't just a passive passenger. It also exhibits **unique chemical interactions** with other molecules. It can form weak bonds with solutes, stabilizing them and enhancing their absorption. This is why DMSO is often used in combination with other therapeutic agents; it acts as a vehicle, increasing their bioavailability.

Another noteworthy characteristic is DMSO's role as an **antioxidant**. It can scavenge free radicals—unstable molecules that can damage cells and contribute to aging and disease. By neutralizing these free radicals, DMSO helps protect cells from oxidative stress.

Furthermore, DMSO has a high **boiling point** (189°C or 372°F) and a low **freezing point** (18.5°C or 65°F), which is why it sometimes crystallizes at room temperature, especially in cooler climates. If you find your DMSO has turned solid, don't worry—it's still perfectly good. Gently warming the container in warm (not hot) water will return it to liquid form without degrading its quality.

It's also worth mentioning that DMSO is **hygroscopic**, meaning it readily absorbs water from the environment. This property underscores the importance of keeping your DMSO in a well-sealed container to maintain its purity and efficacy.

Now, let's touch on the **safety aspect** of DMSO's chemistry. Because it can carry other substances through the skin and into the bloodstream, it's crucial to ensure that anything coming into contact with DMSO is pure and non-toxic. This includes the surfaces it touches, the containers it's stored in (glass is preferred), and the tools used for application.

In summary, the uniqueness of DMSO lies in its:

- **Polar aprotic nature**: Allows it to dissolve a wide range of substances.
- **Transdermal penetration**: Enables it to carry therapeutic agents deep into tissues.
- **Antioxidant properties**: Protects cells from oxidative damage.
- **Chemical stability**: Maintains its integrity under various conditions.

Understanding these properties isn't just an academic exercise; it's the key to unlocking DMSO's full potential. Whether you're formulating a remedy for joint pain or exploring skin rejuvenation techniques, knowing how DMSO interacts on a molecular level will help you make informed choices and achieve better results.

As we move forward, we'll build on this foundation, exploring practical applications and recipes that harness these unique chemical characteristics. Remember, knowledge is power, and in the case of DMSO, it's the bridge between curiosity and confident, effective use.

1.3 The Multitasking Molecule: Properties and Mechanisms

A Born Problem Solver

At first glance, DMSO's molecular structure—simple, small, and efficient—doesn't seem remarkable. But it's in this simplicity that its genius lies. With two methyl groups and a sulfur-oxygen bond, DMSO operates with the precision of a master craftsman. It can slip through the skin and cellular membranes like a thread through a needle, carrying other substances along for the ride. This ability to penetrate tissue without causing harm is one of the reasons it has captivated scientists for decades.

Take, for instance, its use as a carrier molecule. If you've ever applied a cream or lotion, you know that most of it lingers on the skin's surface. DMSO, however, doesn't stop there—it dives deeper, delivering therapeutic agents directly to the cells that need them. Whether it's magnesium for muscle relief or turmeric for inflammation, DMSO enhances their bioavailability, ensuring they're absorbed efficiently.

Inflammation's Worst Enemy

Inflammation is at the root of countless health issues, from swollen joints to chronic disease. What makes DMSO such a powerful anti-inflammatory is its ability to calm the storm at the cellular level. Picture a firefighter dousing flames—DMSO stabilizes cell membranes, preventing them from releasing inflammatory signals like prostaglandins and cytokines. It's like putting out the fire before it spreads, making it invaluable for conditions like arthritis, tendonitis, and sports injuries.

A Fast-Acting Pain Reliever

If you've ever winced from a sharp pain or endured the dull ache of a chronic condition, you know how relentless discomfort can be. DMSO acts as a natural anesthetic, blocking nerve signals and providing almost immediate relief. But it doesn't stop there—by reducing inflammation, it tackles the underlying cause of pain, offering both short-term comfort and long-term healing. This dual action is why it's trusted by athletes, physical therapists, and everyday users alike.

A Shield Against Oxidative Stress

Every day, our bodies face an invisible threat: oxidative stress. Caused by free radicals, these unstable molecules damage cells, accelerate aging, and contribute to chronic diseases. DMSO is a potent antioxidant, neutralizing these free radicals and protecting your cells like a suit of armor. This isn't just theory—it's been demonstrated in studies where DMSO's antioxidant properties reduced damage in conditions ranging from cardiovascular issues to neurodegenerative diseases.

The Circulation Enhancer

DMSO doesn't just work on a cellular level—it also improves how your body delivers nutrients and removes waste. As a vasodilator, it widens blood vessels, increasing circulation to tissues in need. Imagine a delivery truck reaching every corner of the city faster and more efficiently. By enhancing blood flow, DMSO speeds up recovery, reduces swelling, and promotes overall healing.

A Friend to Cryopreservation

DMSO's journey into the medical world includes an unexpected detour into cryopreservation—the process of freezing biological samples like stem cells and embryos. When cells are frozen, ice crystals can form, causing irreversible damage. DMSO prevents this by stabilizing cell membranes, ensuring that the samples remain viable even after years in storage. It's this same protective mechanism that underscores DMSO's value in preserving not just cells, but health.

Crossing Boundaries—Literally

Few substances can cross the blood-brain barrier, the body's natural defense that protects the brain from harmful agents. DMSO is one of the rare exceptions. This ability has sparked interest in its potential for treating brain injuries, reducing swelling, and even delivering medications directly to the central nervous system. While research in this area is ongoing, the implications are profound.

A Natural Antimicrobial

Though not its primary function, DMSO has been shown to inhibit the growth of certain bacteria, viruses, and fungi. This adds another layer to its usefulness, particularly in wound care and infection management. Combined with its anti-inflammatory and circulation-enhancing properties, it's a natural ally for supporting the body's defenses.

Bringing It All Together

DMSO's true brilliance lies in how its properties complement one another. Its anti-inflammatory effects reduce swelling, its pain-relieving action brings comfort, and its carrier ability ensures that other therapeutic agents reach their target. Add to this its antioxidant and vasodilatory roles, and you have a molecule that works in harmony with the body's natural processes.

But with great power comes great responsibility. DMSO's ability to penetrate deeply means that cleanliness and quality are non-negotiable. The tools you use, the skin you apply it to, and the substances it interacts with must be pure and safe. This isn't just about maximizing benefits—it's about protecting yourself from unintended consequences.

DMSO is more than a chemical—it's a partner in healing. Whether you're using it for pain relief, recovery, or holistic wellness, its multitasking nature offers endless possibilities. Its ability to adapt to so many roles is a testament to its chemistry, and to the idea that some solutions—though simple on the surface—are profoundly complex in their potential.

Chapter 2

THE EVOLUTION OF DMSO

2.1 Historical Uses Across Industries

The story of DMSO begins in an unexpected place—not in a medical lab or a natural remedy handbook, but in the industrial yards of 19th-century Europe. Picture it: large factories churning out paper, workers surrounded by mountains of wood pulp, and amidst it all, a curious byproduct trickling away in the background. This unassuming liquid, extracted during the process of breaking down lignin—the tough polymer that gives plants their rigidity—was DMSO.

In its early days, DMSO was little more than a solvent, valued for its ability to dissolve both organic and inorganic materials. Industrial chemists quickly realized that it was unmatched in its versatility. From cleaning machinery to aiding in chemical reactions, it became a workhorse in industries as diverse as manufacturing, textiles, and petroleum refining. For decades, it lived in the shadows, a reliable but unremarkable player in the industrial world.

But like any good story, DMSO's journey took a surprising turn.

The First Glimpse of Something More

In the early 20th century, a few curious scientists began to wonder if this powerful solvent had uses beyond the factory floor. Its ability to penetrate surfaces fascinated them, as did its apparent lack of toxicity. Could it be something more than just a cleaner or dissolver? These early inklings planted the seeds for what would later become a full-blown scientific exploration.

World War II brought with it a flurry of research and innovation, and DMSO found a new role in the war effort. It was used to preserve and transport chemical agents, thanks to its stability and compatibility with a wide range of substances. Soldiers and medics also discovered its ability to reduce frostbite in freezing conditions—a clue to its potential for protecting human tissues.

The Medical Awakening

The real breakthrough came in the 1960s when Dr. Stanley Jacob, a surgeon at the University of Oregon, stumbled across DMSO while searching for ways to preserve organs for transplantation. What he found was far more intriguing: not only did DMSO prevent ice crystals from forming in cells during freezing, but it also seemed to have profound biological effects. It reduced inflammation, eased pain, and, most fascinatingly, carried other substances directly through the skin and into the bloodstream.

Dr. Jacob's discovery sparked a wave of excitement—and controversy. Suddenly, this industrial solvent was being touted as a potential medical marvel. Researchers rushed to study its effects on everything from arthritis to sports injuries, and anecdotal reports of its healing properties began to pour in. Yet, for every enthusiastic endorsement, there was skepticism. Could something so versatile really be safe? And why did it make people smell faintly of garlic?

Beyond Medicine: Expanding the Horizon

Even as DMSO's medical potential became a hot topic, its uses in other industries continued to expand. In agriculture, it became a trusted ally for delivering nutrients and pesticides directly into plant tissues. Veterinary medicine adopted it for treating joint and muscle injuries in horses and other animals. And in cryopreservation, it became indispensable for freezing and storing biological samples like stem cells, embryos, and blood.

The scientific community marveled at DMSO's adaptability. Here was a compound that could clean an engine, preserve a cell, and ease a sprained ankle—all with equal effectiveness. Yet, its industrial origins and "too good to be true" reputation often worked against it. Regulatory agencies hesitated, public perceptions wavered, and DMSO remained a misunderstood enigma.

A Symbol of Untapped Potential

Today, looking back at DMSO's evolution, one thing is clear: its story is far from over. What began as a simple byproduct of the paper industry has become a symbol of untapped potential—a reminder that even the most unassuming substances can hold extraordinary power.

As we move forward in this chapter, we'll delve deeper into the challenges and triumphs that shaped DMSO's journey, exploring how it transitioned from factory floors to clinics, and ultimately, to the hands of people like you and me. Its history isn't just a tale of science and innovation; it's a testament to curiosity, persistence, and the human drive to discover.

2.2 Pioneering Medical Applications

DMSO's transition from industrial solvent to medical marvel was anything but conventional. In the mid-20th century, researchers were beginning to explore the boundaries of what this unassuming molecule could do. Among them was Dr. Stanley Jacob, a surgeon at the University of Oregon, whose work would forever change the trajectory of DMSO and its place in modern medicine.

The Unexpected Discovery

It was the 1960s, and Dr. Jacob was searching for a way to improve organ preservation for transplants. At the time, one of the biggest challenges in transplant medicine was preventing ice crystals from forming inside cells during freezing. These microscopic shards would rupture cell membranes, rendering organs unusable. Enter DMSO. As an industrial solvent, it was known for its ability to stabilize compounds under extreme conditions. When Dr. Jacob tested it, he found that DMSO could protect cells during freezing, preserving their integrity and opening new possibilities for organ storage.

But this was only the beginning.

While experimenting with DMSO, Dr. Jacob noticed something remarkable: patients reported a reduction in pain and swelling near the application site. Intrigued, he began to investigate its potential beyond cryopreservation. What he discovered was nothing short of groundbreaking—a compound that could reduce inflammation, alleviate pain, and carry other substances through the skin and into the bloodstream.

A Medical Renaissance

The medical community was electrified by DMSO's potential. Here was a substance that seemed to do it all. It wasn't just an anti-inflammatory; it was a pain reliever, a carrier molecule, and even a possible treatment for certain chronic conditions. Clinical trials sprang up around the world, testing DMSO for everything from arthritis to sports injuries.

One of the most notable studies came out of Russia, where researchers had already been using DMSO to treat burns and skin conditions. They found that it accelerated wound healing, reduced scarring, and minimized pain. Across the Atlantic, American scientists were uncovering similar results. For people with arthritis, applying DMSO to swollen joints offered relief that traditional treatments couldn't match. Athletes turned to it for faster recovery from injuries, while dermatologists explored its potential for treating skin conditions like psoriasis and eczema.

A Polarizing Substance

As DMSO gained traction, it also garnered controversy. The same properties that made it so promising—its ability to penetrate skin and transport substances—raised red flags for regulators. Could DMSO inadvertently carry harmful chemicals into the body? Were there long-term risks that hadn't yet been studied? And what about the infamous garlic-like odor it left on users' breath, a harmless but stigmatizing side effect that made skeptics scoff?

In 1965, the U.S. Food and Drug Administration (FDA) approved DMSO for clinical trials, but its momentum was soon slowed by concerns over toxicity and inconsistent results in some studies. The FDA eventually approved DMSO for treating interstitial cystitis, a painful bladder condition, but hesitated to greenlight broader applications. Meanwhile, patients and practitioners who had experienced its benefits continued to advocate for its wider use, fueling a divide between conventional medicine and alternative health communities.

Breaking New Ground

Despite these hurdles, DMSO found its champions in both human and veterinary medicine. Doctors used it off-label to treat conditions like scleroderma, a rare autoimmune disease that causes hardening of the skin and connective tissues. Veterinarians embraced it for treating lameness and inflammation in horses, where its ability to penetrate thick tissue was especially valuable. Its use in sports medicine also flourished, with trainers relying on DMSO to keep athletes in peak condition.

But DMSO's influence wasn't limited to clinical settings. It became a symbol of innovation, a reminder that nature often holds solutions we're only beginning to understand. Researchers continued to explore its potential, studying its effects on neurological conditions, cardiovascular health, and even cancer. While some findings were preliminary, they hinted at a future where DMSO could play a key role in treating some of the most challenging diseases.

A Legacy of Curiosity

The journey of DMSO from industrial solvent to medical tool is a testament to the power of curiosity and persistence. What began as a chance discovery during organ preservation experiments evolved into a global exploration of one of nature's most versatile compounds. Along the way, DMSO faced challenges, skeptics, and regulatory roadblocks. But it also inspired a community of scientists, doctors, and everyday users who saw its potential and refused to let it be forgotten.

Today, DMSO continues to straddle the line between mainstream medicine and holistic health. Its history reminds us that some of the most profound breakthroughs come from asking simple questions: What else can this do? How can we make it better? And what possibilities might we unlock if we're willing to look beyond the surface?

As we continue this chapter, we'll delve deeper into the triumphs and trials that have defined DMSO's evolution, exploring how it has shaped—and been shaped by—the people who believed in its promise.

2.3 The Controversy and FDA Regulation

Every innovation that challenges convention inevitably faces resistance, and DMSO is no exception. For all its promise, this remarkable compound has spent much of its history at the center of heated debates, regulatory scrutiny, and public misunderstanding. Its journey through the corridors of approval is a story of hope, caution, and the clash between innovation and the status quo.

The Surge of Excitement

The 1960s marked the golden era of DMSO's rise in medicine. With researchers like Dr. Stanley Jacob leading the charge, studies poured in showcasing its potential as a pain reliever, anti-inflammatory, and carrier molecule. Patients raved about its ability to ease arthritis pain, accelerate healing, and improve mobility. For a moment, it seemed as though DMSO was destined to revolutionize healthcare.

But with great attention comes great scrutiny. As DMSO captured headlines and drew the interest of both the medical community and the public, questions about its safety began to emerge. Its ability to carry substances through the skin, while groundbreaking, raised concerns about what else it might transport—chemicals, toxins, or harmful contaminants. Could this same property that made DMSO so versatile also make it dangerous?

The Infamous Trials

The turning point came in 1965, when the FDA approved DMSO for clinical trials in the United States. It was a significant step forward, fueled by promising research and public demand. However, the trials quickly became a double-edged sword.

Some participants experienced side effects, most notably changes in their vision and the infamous garlic-like odor on their breath—a harmless but unpleasant byproduct of DMSO's metabolism. While these effects were relatively mild, they added fuel to skeptics who questioned the compound's safety. Compounding the issue were inconsistencies in the study results. While some trials demonstrated clear benefits, others were inconclusive, leading to confusion and hesitation among regulators.

By the late 1960s, the FDA had tightened its stance. Though it didn't outright ban DMSO, it severely limited its approved uses, citing insufficient evidence of safety and efficacy. The only official approval granted was for the treatment of interstitial cystitis, a painful bladder condition that had few other effective therapies at the time. For proponents of DMSO, it was a frustrating setback. For critics, it was validation of their concerns.

Public Perception and Stigma

The FDA's cautious approach reverberated beyond the medical community. News outlets, eager for a sensational story, seized on the narrative of DMSO as a controversial, misunderstood remedy. Headlines emphasized its industrial origins and side effects, while downplaying its potential benefits. Public opinion began to shift, and DMSO became a polarizing topic. For every patient who swore by its healing properties, there was someone else dismissing it as snake oil.

Adding to the stigma was DMSO's association with alternative medicine. As its use became more restricted in mainstream healthcare, it found a home in holistic and natural health circles. While this allowed DMSO to thrive among those who valued its accessibility and effectiveness, it also widened the gap between proponents and detractors. For many in conventional medicine, DMSO became a cautionary tale—a reminder of what happens when enthusiasm outpaces evidence.

Behind the Scenes: The Politics of Regulation

What often gets lost in the story of DMSO is the broader context of medical regulation. The FDA's cautious stance wasn't just about DMSO—it reflected the agency's evolving role in safeguarding public health during a time of rapid scientific advancement. In the wake of tragedies like the thalidomide crisis, where insufficient testing led to catastrophic birth defects, the FDA faced immense pressure to prioritize safety above all else. DMSO, with its complex mechanisms and multifaceted effects, presented a regulatory challenge that didn't fit neatly into the frameworks of the time.

Moreover, the pharmaceutical industry played a subtle but significant role in shaping the narrative. Unlike patented drugs, DMSO was a naturally occurring substance that couldn't be easily commercialized. Without the backing of major pharmaceutical companies, it lacked the financial and institutional support needed to navigate the lengthy and expensive approval process. This dynamic further complicated its journey, as skeptics pointed to its lack of industry endorsement as a red flag, while proponents saw it as evidence of systemic bias against natural remedies.

A Second Wave of Interest

Despite these challenges, DMSO's story didn't end in the 1960s. Over the decades, renewed interest in natural and alternative therapies has brought it back into the spotlight. Modern research has begun to validate many of the claims made by its early advocates, and practitioners in fields like sports medicine, dermatology, and veterinary care continue to use it with success.

The FDA has also softened its stance somewhat, allowing for expanded research into DMSO's applications. While its approval remains limited, its use off-label and in holistic health practices has ensured that it remains a vital tool for those willing to explore its potential.

A Legacy of Controversy and Hope

The controversy surrounding DMSO is a reminder of the complexities of innovation in healthcare. Balancing safety, efficacy, and accessibility is no small feat, especially for a substance as multifaceted as this one. Yet, for all its challenges, DMSO's story is ultimately one of resilience. It has survived regulatory hurdles, public skepticism, and shifting medical paradigms to remain a powerful, if underappreciated, ally in the pursuit of healing.

As we move forward in this chapter, we'll explore how DMSO has navigated these obstacles to become a symbol of both controversy and possibility—a testament to the enduring power of discovery and the courage to challenge the norm.

2.4 DMSO Today: Approved and Off-Label Uses

DMSO's story didn't end with regulatory hurdles and public skepticism. In fact, those chapters merely set the stage for its enduring role in modern medicine and holistic health. Today, DMSO occupies a fascinating space: officially sanctioned for a narrow range of medical applications but widely embraced for an array of off-label uses that continue to expand its reputation as a versatile and invaluable compound.

What the FDA Approves

For all its multifaceted potential, DMSO's official uses in the United States remain limited. Since the 1970s, the FDA has approved DMSO primarily for the treatment of **interstitial cystitis**, a chronic bladder condition characterized by inflammation and intense pain. For many patients with interstitial cystitis, DMSO has been a lifeline, providing relief where other treatments have failed. Delivered directly into the bladder via catheter, it reduces inflammation, relieves discomfort, and improves overall quality of life.

In veterinary medicine, DMSO has also gained official recognition, particularly for its use in treating lameness and swelling in horses. Its ability to penetrate thick tissue and deliver therapeutic effects deep into joints and muscles has made it a favorite among equine practitioners.

But beyond these sanctioned uses lies a far broader story—one shaped by the creativity and determination of practitioners, researchers, and individuals who have explored DMSO's untapped potential.

Off-Label and Alternative Applications

Ask a seasoned natural health practitioner about DMSO, and you'll likely hear a long list of its off-label uses. While these applications lack formal FDA approval, they are supported by anecdotal evidence, preliminary studies, and decades of practical experience.

1. **Pain Relief**

    One of DMSO's most celebrated uses is for managing pain. Whether it's applied to aching joints, sore muscles, or nerve-related discomfort, its ability to penetrate tissues and block pain signals makes it an invaluable tool for many. Athletes often turn to DMSO for rapid recovery from sports injuries, while people with chronic pain conditions like arthritis or fibromyalgia find it offers relief without the side effects of traditional painkillers.

2. **Skin and Wound Healing**

    DMSO's antimicrobial, anti-inflammatory, and circulation-enhancing properties make it a natural choice for treating cuts, burns, and other skin injuries. Some users swear by it for reducing scarring, soothing eczema, or calming psoriasis flare-ups. Its ability to carry healing agents like aloe vera or essential oils deeper into the skin amplifies its effectiveness.

3. **Anti-Inflammatory Uses**

    Inflammation lies at the heart of many chronic conditions, from autoimmune disorders to cardiovascular diseases. By stabilizing cell membranes and reducing inflammatory mediators, DMSO has been used off-label to manage conditions like tendonitis, bursitis, and even inflammatory bowel disease.

4. Neurological Conditions

   DMSO's ability to cross the blood-brain barrier has sparked interest in its potential for neurological applications. While still in the early stages of research, some practitioners have explored its use in managing conditions like traumatic brain injuries, multiple sclerosis, and even Alzheimer's disease. These applications remain experimental but represent a promising frontier.

5. Detoxification and Heavy Metal Chelation

   In holistic health circles, DMSO is often used as part of detoxification protocols. Its ability to bind with toxins and transport them out of the body has made it a favorite for those seeking to reduce heavy metal buildup or support overall cellular health. When paired with agents like activated charcoal or bentonite clay, DMSO's detoxifying effects are amplified.

6. Cryopreservation

   Beyond therapeutic applications, DMSO continues to play a critical role in the preservation of biological materials. Its ability to protect cells from damage during freezing has made it indispensable for storing stem cells, embryos, and other biological samples in research and medicine.

A Tool for Holistic and Integrative Medicine

What makes DMSO particularly compelling today is its dual role in both conventional and alternative medicine. In integrative health practices, it's often paired with complementary therapies like acupuncture, herbal remedies, or dietary protocols. This holistic approach maximizes its benefits while addressing the root causes of health challenges.

For many, DMSO represents a bridge—a way to combine the best of modern science with the wisdom of natural healing. Its affordability and accessibility mean that it's not confined to the realm of high-cost pharmaceuticals. Instead, it's a tool that empowers individuals to take an active role in their health.

The Ongoing Exploration

The story of DMSO is still being written. Researchers continue to investigate its potential for new applications, from cancer treatment to cardiovascular health. Meanwhile, everyday users and practitioners contribute to its evolving legacy, sharing their experiences and expanding its possibilities.

What remains consistent is the core principle that defines DMSO: it works with the body, not against it. Whether you're addressing a chronic condition, seeking faster recovery, or exploring preventative care, DMSO offers a natural, science-backed solution that adapts to your needs.

As we close this chapter, one thing becomes clear: DMSO's greatest strength isn't just its versatility—it's its ability to inspire curiosity, innovation, and hope. From its approved uses to its off-label applications, DMSO continues to defy expectations, reminding us that even the simplest compounds can unlock profound healing.

Part II

SAFE USE AND PREPARATION

CHAPTER 3

PREPARING TO USE DMSO

3.1 Selecting the Right Product: Pharmaceutical vs. Industrial Grades

Choosing the right DMSO product is the first and most crucial step in your journey. With its diverse applications across industries, not all DMSO is created equal, and understanding the differences can mean the difference between a safe, effective experience and potential complications. Let's dive into what sets DMSO products apart and how to select one that meets your needs.

From Factory Floors to First Aid Kits

DMSO originated as an industrial solvent, and many of its products still cater to that purpose. In manufacturing, it's used to clean machinery, extract chemicals, and act as a medium for reactions. But the same chemical that can cut through industrial grime is not what you want on your skin—or in your body.

This is where the distinction between **industrial-grade** and **pharmaceutical-grade** DMSO becomes critical. While the core compound is the same, the processing, purity, and intended use of these products differ significantly.

Industrial-Grade DMSO: The Workhorse

Industrial-grade DMSO is the version most commonly used in factories and laboratories. It's robust, effective, and cost-efficient, but it's not intended for human or veterinary use. Here's why:

- **Purity Concerns**: Industrial-grade DMSO often contains impurities, byproducts, or residual solvents from manufacturing processes. While these impurities may not matter in industrial applications, they can pose serious risks when applied to the body.
- **Storage Standards**: Industrial DMSO is typically stored in plastic containers that aren't designed to meet medical-grade cleanliness standards. Given DMSO's ability to leach chemicals from plastics, this raises red flags for safety.
- **Regulatory Oversight**: Industrial-grade products are not subject to the rigorous testing and quality controls required for pharmaceutical-grade substances.

While it may be tempting to save money by purchasing industrial-grade DMSO, the risks far outweigh the benefits. Your health is worth investing in a product designed for therapeutic use.

Pharmaceutical-Grade DMSO: The Healer

Pharmaceutical-grade DMSO is held to much higher standards. It is purified, tested, and manufactured with medical and therapeutic applications in mind. Here's what sets it apart:

- **Purity**: Pharmaceutical-grade DMSO is typically **99.9% pure**, meaning it contains virtually no contaminants or byproducts. This level of purity ensures that the DMSO is safe for transdermal (skin) application and internal use when recommended by a practitioner.
- **Packaging**: Medical-grade DMSO is often stored in glass containers to prevent leaching or contamination. This is particularly important given DMSO's ability to absorb impurities.
- **Testing and Regulation**: Pharmaceutical-grade products undergo rigorous testing for safety, potency, and consistency. While regulations vary by country, reputable brands ensure their products meet the highest standards.

If you're planning to use DMSO for therapeutic purposes—whether it's for pain relief, inflammation, or skin health—pharmaceutical-grade is the only way to go.

Reading the Label: What to Look For

When purchasing DMSO, the label holds the key to ensuring you're getting a safe product. Here are the essential details to check:

1. **Purity**: Look for products labeled as **99.9% pure** or higher. Anything less may contain impurities that could be harmful.
2. **Grade**: Ensure the label specifies **pharmaceutical-grade** or **medical-grade**. If it says "industrial-grade," it's not suitable for therapeutic use.

3. **Packaging**: Opt for products stored in glass bottles. Avoid plastic containers, as DMSO can leach chemicals from plastics.
4. **Manufacturer Reputation**: Choose a product from a reputable brand with clear sourcing and quality control practices. Online reviews and third-party certifications can help guide your decision.

Red Flags to Avoid

Even with a plethora of options on the market, not all products are trustworthy. Watch out for these warning signs:

- **Vague Labeling**: If the label doesn't specify purity or grade, steer clear.
- **Unsealed Packaging**: Properly sealed bottles are crucial for maintaining purity.
- **Suspiciously Low Prices**: If a product seems too good to be true, it likely is. High-quality DMSO reflects its rigorous production process in its price.

Where to Buy High-Quality DMSO

Pharmaceutical-grade DMSO is widely available online and through specialized health retailers. Reputable sources include:

- **Health Stores**: Many natural health stores carry pharmaceutical-grade DMSO.
- **Online Retailers**: Websites specializing in alternative medicine or wellness products often stock DMSO. Look for transparent labeling and verified reviews.
- **Compounding Pharmacies**: In some cases, pharmacies that prepare custom medications may also supply high-quality DMSO.

A Final Word on Quality

When it comes to DMSO, quality isn't just important—it's non-negotiable. Choosing a pharmaceutical-grade product ensures that you're using a safe, effective substance designed for therapeutic use. By taking the time to understand the differences between grades and selecting a reputable source, you're setting the foundation for a successful and empowering DMSO experience.

As we move forward in this chapter, we'll explore how to prepare, store, and use your DMSO safely and effectively, ensuring that you get the most out of this incredible compound.

3.2 Dilution Charts and Mixing Ratios

One of the most critical aspects of using DMSO safely and effectively is understanding how to dilute it. Whether you're applying it to your skin, using it as part of a remedy, or preparing it for a specific condition, proper dilution is essential. The good news? It's easier than you think. With a bit of guidance and a reliable dilution chart, you'll have everything you need to create solutions tailored to your needs.

Why Dilution Matters

DMSO in its pure form—99.9% pharmaceutical-grade—is incredibly potent. While this purity ensures that the product is free from contaminants, applying DMSO at full strength is rarely recommended. Here's why dilution is so important:

1. **Skin Sensitivity**: Undiluted DMSO can cause irritation, redness, or a burning sensation, especially on sensitive skin.

2. **Controlled Absorption**: Diluting DMSO allows you to control how much of the compound (and any accompanying substances) is absorbed by your body.
3. **Customizability**: Different conditions and application areas require different strengths. Dilution gives you the flexibility to tailor solutions for specific needs.

Understanding Dilution Percentages

Dilution percentages refer to the proportion of DMSO to distilled water in your solution. For example, a 50% dilution means equal parts DMSO and water, while a 70% dilution contains 70% DMSO and 30% water.

Here's a quick guide to common dilution levels and their uses:

Dilution Percentage	Common Uses	Sensitivity
90%	Severe joint pain, thick skin areas (e.g., knees, elbows)	Low sensitivity areas
70%	General pain relief, inflammation, arthritis	Moderate sensitivity
50%	Delicate skin, chronic conditions, general use	High sensitivity
30%	Facial applications, highly sensitive skin	Extremely delicate

Note: For internal or advanced applications, always consult a professional.

Step-by-Step Guide to Mixing DMSO

Making your own DMSO solution is simple, but precision is key. Follow these steps to ensure a safe and effective dilution:

What You'll Need

- Pharmaceutical-grade DMSO (99.9% pure)
- Distilled water (not tap water, to avoid impurities)
- Glass measuring cups or syringes (avoid plastic, as DMSO can leach chemicals from it)
- A clean glass container with a secure lid for storage

How to Mix

1. **Determine Your Desired Dilution**: Decide on the percentage of DMSO you need based on the application.
2. **Measure Your Ingredients**:
    - For a 70% solution: Combine 7 parts DMSO with 3 parts distilled water.
    - For a 50% solution: Mix equal parts DMSO and distilled water.
    - For a 30% solution: Use 3 parts DMSO and 7 parts water.
3. **Combine and Mix**: Pour the measured DMSO and water into a clean glass container. Stir gently with a glass or stainless-steel utensil to ensure the solution is evenly mixed.
4. **Label Your Solution**: Clearly mark the container with the dilution percentage and the date of preparation.
5. **Store Safely**: Keep your solution in a cool, dark place, ideally in an amber glass bottle to protect it from light and contamination.

Troubleshooting and Tips

Even with precise measurements, you might encounter some common issues when mixing DMSO. Here's how to address them:

- **Cloudy Solution**: This may occur if tap water or impure distilled water is used. Always opt for high-quality distilled water to prevent this.
- **Crystallization**: If your solution crystallizes at cooler temperatures, gently warm the bottle in lukewarm water. Avoid overheating, as this can degrade the DMSO.
- **Sticky Texture**: If your solution feels sticky, you may have used too much DMSO. Adjust by adding more water to achieve the desired consistency.

Practical Applications

Here's a breakdown of how different dilutions can be used in practice:

- **90%**: Ideal for thick skin areas like knees or elbows, especially for severe joint pain or inflammation.
- **70%**: The go-to dilution for most applications, including back pain, arthritis, and moderate inflammation.
- **50%**: Best for beginners or those with sensitive skin, offering a balanced concentration for general use.
- **30%**: Perfect for facial applications or delicate areas like the neck and inner arms.

Charts for Quick Reference

To make things even simpler, here's a quick-reference table for commonly used dilutions:

Desired Dilution	Parts DMSO	Parts Water	Example (10 mL)
90%	9	1	9 mL DMSO + 1 mL water
70%	7	3	7 mL DMSO + 3 mL water
50%	1	1	5 mL DMSO + 5 mL water
30%	3	7	3 mL DMSO + 7 mL water

A Word on Safety

Always prioritize safety when working with DMSO. Use clean, high-quality tools, store your solutions properly, and remember that dilution isn't just about effectiveness—it's about protecting your skin and body from unnecessary irritation or harm.

As we move forward, we'll explore the tools and techniques you'll need to apply your DMSO solutions effectively, ensuring that you can harness the full power of this incredible compound.

3.3 Tools and Equipment for Safe Application

DMSO is a versatile compound, but its powerful properties mean that the tools and equipment you use can make or break your experience. Whether you're mixing solutions, applying DMSO to your skin, or storing it for future use, having the right tools isn't just a matter of convenience—it's essential for safety and effectiveness.

The Essentials of Working with DMSO

DMSO's ability to penetrate surfaces and carry substances into the body means that every tool it touches must be carefully chosen. Here's why: DMSO doesn't discriminate. If it comes into contact with plastic, impurities, or contaminants, it can carry those unwanted substances right into your skin and bloodstream. That's why using clean, compatible, and high-quality tools is non-negotiable.

What You'll Need

Here's a breakdown of the must-have tools for working with DMSO, along with tips for choosing the best options:

1. Measuring Tools

- **Why They Matter**: Accurate measurements are key when mixing DMSO solutions. Too much DMSO can cause irritation, while too little may reduce its effectiveness.
- **What to Use**:
  - Glass measuring cups or syringes for precise measurements.
  - Avoid plastic measuring tools, as DMSO can degrade certain plastics and leach chemicals.
- **Pro Tip**: Look for glass syringes with clear volume markings for smaller quantities.

2. Mixing Utensils

- **Why They Matter**: Ensuring a consistent solution requires proper mixing.
- **What to Use**:
  - Glass stir rods or stainless-steel utensils.

- Avoid wooden or plastic utensils, as they can absorb or react with DMSO.
- **Pro Tip**: Keep dedicated tools for DMSO to avoid cross-contamination.

3. Storage Containers

- **Why They Matter**: DMSO is hygroscopic, meaning it absorbs moisture from the air. Improper storage can compromise its purity and effectiveness.
- **What to Use**:
  - Amber or dark glass bottles with airtight seals to protect from light and air exposure.
  - Avoid plastic containers, as DMSO can leach harmful chemicals.
- **Pro Tip**: Label your containers with the dilution percentage and date of preparation for easy reference.

4. Applicators

- **Why They Matter**: Applying DMSO requires precision to ensure even coverage without contamination.
- **What to Use**:
  - Cotton balls, gauze pads, or natural fiber brushes for direct application.
  - Silicone applicators are safe for certain uses, but always check compatibility.
  - Avoid synthetic sponges or applicators made of unknown materials.
- **Pro Tip**: Discard used applicators after each session to maintain hygiene.

5. **Protective Gear**

- **Why It Matters**: While DMSO is safe when used correctly, protective gear can prevent accidental exposure or irritation.
- **What to Use**:
    - Nitrile or latex gloves to protect your hands.
    - Protective eyewear if you're handling larger quantities.
- **Pro Tip**: Choose gloves free of powders or additives to avoid transferring impurities.

Setting Up Your Workspace

A clean and organized workspace ensures that your DMSO experience is safe and efficient. Here's how to create the perfect setup:

1. **Choose a Flat, Stable Surface**: Prevent spills and accidents by working on a level table or countertop.
2. **Cover Your Work Area**: Use a clean, disposable cloth or a silicone mat to protect your surface.
3. **Keep It Minimal**: Limit the tools and items in your workspace to reduce the risk of contamination.
4. **Ensure Ventilation**: While DMSO doesn't produce harmful fumes, a well-ventilated area is always a good idea.

Cleaning and Maintaining Your Tools

DMSO is reusable-friendly, but cleaning your tools after each use is vital to avoid contamination. Here's a quick guide:

- **Step 1**: Rinse tools immediately after use with distilled water to remove residue.

- **Step 2**: Wash with a mild, fragrance-free soap, using a soft sponge or cloth.
- **Step 3**: Rinse thoroughly with distilled water to ensure no soap or residue remains.
- **Step 4**: Allow tools to air dry completely before storing or reusing.

Common Mistakes to Avoid

Even seasoned users can make errors when working with DMSO. Here's what to watch out for:

- **Using Plastic Tools**: DMSO's ability to leach chemicals from plastic makes this a major no-no.
- **Reusing Dirty Applicators**: Always use fresh cotton balls or gauze to avoid reintroducing impurities.
- **Eyeballing Measurements**: Accurate mixing is crucial for safety and effectiveness. Always measure carefully.
- **Improvised Storage**: Resist the temptation to store DMSO in leftover jars or containers. Stick to properly sealed glass bottles.

Where to Source Quality Tools

High-quality tools are widely available and don't have to break the bank. Here are a few places to find what you need:

- **Health Stores**: Many carry glass measuring tools, syringes, and applicators suitable for DMSO.
- **Online Retailers**: Websites specializing in holistic health or laboratory equipment often offer a wide range of compatible tools.
- **Local Pharmacies**: For items like glass syringes or nitrile gloves, check with your nearest pharmacy.

A Foundation for Success

The tools you use when working with DMSO aren't just accessories—they're a vital part of your success. By investing in high-quality equipment and taking the time to maintain it, you're ensuring that every application of DMSO is safe, effective, and frustration-free.

As we move to the next section, we'll explore how to set up your workspace and prepare for a seamless DMSO experience, building on the foundation of tools and techniques you've just learned.

3.4 Setting Up a Clean Workspace

When working with DMSO, your workspace isn't just a convenience—it's the foundation of safe and effective use. A clean, organized setup minimizes contamination risks and ensures everything runs smoothly. Setting up a dedicated space is simple, practical, and worth the effort.

Why It Matters

DMSO is a powerhouse at absorbing and transporting substances, but that means it's not picky about what it picks up. Dust, oils, or residue from a surface can end up in your solution—or worse, in your body. A clean workspace is your first line of defense.

Setting Up Your Space

1. Choose a Spot

- Use a flat, stable surface like a table or countertop.
- Avoid areas with food, clutter, or household chemicals.

2. Protect the Surface

- Place a silicone mat, paper towels, or a glass tray to catch spills and keep things tidy.

3. Organize Your Tools

- Keep DMSO-specific items—like syringes, gloves, and applicators—separate from other supplies.
- Use small containers or trays to keep everything in easy reach.

Hygiene Basics

- **Wipe Down Before and After**: Use a mild disinfectant or distilled water to clean your workspace.
- **Wash Your Hands**: A quick scrub with soap and water keeps unwanted oils or dirt out of the mix.
- **Use Fresh Supplies**: Cotton balls, gauze, and applicators should be single-use only.

Ventilation and Storage

- **Airflow**: Crack a window or use a fan if you're working with larger quantities of DMSO.
- **Storage**: Keep DMSO in amber glass bottles, label everything clearly, and store it in a cool, dry place.

Troubleshooting Common Issues

- **Spills**: Clean up immediately with paper towels and distilled water.
- **Clutter**: Keep your setup simple and focused to avoid confusion.

Keep It Simple

A clean workspace doesn't have to be elaborate—just functional and safe. By setting up an organized, dedicated area, you're ensuring that every step of your DMSO journey is as smooth and effective as possible.

Chapter 4

SAFETY AND PRECAUTIONS

4.1 Cleaning and Preparing Skin

When it comes to using DMSO, preparation is everything. Because this compound can carry substances directly through the skin and into the body, ensuring that the application area is clean and ready is a critical step. Think of it like setting the stage for a performance—the better the prep work, the better the results.

Why Preparation Matters

DMSO's ability to penetrate the skin is one of its most powerful features, but it's also what makes preparation so important. Anything lingering on the surface of your skin—dirt, oils, or even unseen residues from soaps and lotions—can hitch a ride with DMSO into your body. That's why a little effort upfront can make a big difference in safety and effectiveness.

Step-by-Step Guide to Preparing Skin

Follow these simple steps to ensure your skin is clean and ready for DMSO application:

1. Wash the Area Thoroughly

- Use warm water and a mild, fragrance-free soap to cleanse the skin. Avoid anything with oils, perfumes, or harsh chemicals, as these can interact with DMSO.
- Rinse well to remove all soap residue.

2. Dry Completely

- Pat the skin dry with a clean, lint-free towel. Make sure the area is completely dry, as moisture can dilute the DMSO or affect absorption.

3. Avoid Contaminants

- Skip lotions, deodorants, or other topical products before applying DMSO. These can mix with the compound and potentially cause irritation or unwanted effects.
- Remove any jewelry or accessories near the application site to prevent interference.

Best Practices for Specific Areas

DMSO can be applied to many areas of the body, but different regions may require slight adjustments in preparation:

- Hands and Arms: Pay extra attention to washing, as these areas often come into contact with various substances throughout the day.

- Joints and Muscles: Clean thoroughly, especially if the area is exposed to sweat or dirt from physical activity.
- Face and Neck: Be gentle, using a soft cloth or your hands to cleanse. Avoid scrubbing, as irritation can increase sensitivity to DMSO.

Common Mistakes to Avoid

Even with the best intentions, it's easy to overlook key steps. Here's what to watch out for:

- Skipping the Wash: Even if the area looks clean, it's essential to wash thoroughly. Invisible residues from soaps, perfumes, or lotions can react with DMSO.
- Using Harsh Products: Avoid anything with alcohol, oils, or strong fragrances. Stick to mild, neutral cleansers.
- Rushing the Process: Take your time to ensure the area is completely clean and dry. A few extra minutes now can save you from potential irritation later.

After Application: Keeping it Clean

Once you've applied DMSO, it's a good idea to maintain a clean environment around the treated area:

- Avoid Touching: Don't touch or rub the area while the DMSO is absorbing, as this can introduce contaminants.
- Rinse After Absorption: After about 20–30 minutes, rinse the area with cool water to remove any residue.

A Simple Routine for Big Results

Cleaning and preparing your skin may feel like a small step, but it's one of the most important things you can do to maximize the benefits of DMSO while minimizing risks. By making it a part of your routine, you're setting yourself up for success—safe, effective, and worry-free.

4.2 Avoiding Contaminants: Why Purity Matters

DMSO's incredible ability to penetrate the skin and carry substances into the body is what makes it so effective—but it's also why purity matters more than anything else. Imagine letting a guest into your home who brings along uninvited companions. That's exactly what contaminants can do when they hitch a ride with DMSO into your system. Let's explore why this matters and how to ensure everything in your DMSO routine stays clean and pure.

The Risks of Contamination

DMSO's transdermal properties mean it doesn't discriminate—it will absorb and transport whatever it encounters. This can include:

- **Dirt and Debris**: Tiny particles from surfaces or the environment can easily mix with your DMSO.
- **Residues**: Lotions, soaps, perfumes, or oils left on the skin can interact with DMSO, potentially causing irritation or unwanted reactions.
- **Plastic Chemicals**: DMSO can leach harmful substances, such as phthalates, from plastic containers or tools.

These contaminants may not seem like a big deal at first glance, but when introduced into your body, they can cause irritation, toxicity, or reduced effectiveness of the DMSO.

How to Avoid Contaminants

The good news? Keeping your DMSO routine clean and contaminant-free is simple with a few mindful steps.

1. Use Pharmaceutical-Grade DMSO

Start with the purest product available. Pharmaceutical-grade DMSO is 99.9% pure and free from the impurities often found in industrial-grade versions. Always check the label and source your DMSO from a reputable supplier.

2. Choose Glass Over Plastic

Store DMSO in amber or clear glass bottles with airtight seals. Plastic containers can leach chemicals into the solution, especially when exposed to heat or light. Glass eliminates this risk while maintaining the integrity of your DMSO.

3. Keep Your Tools Clean

- Use glass or stainless-steel tools for mixing and application.
- Avoid wooden or plastic utensils, as they can harbor contaminants or react with the DMSO.
- Clean your tools with distilled water and a mild soap after each use, and allow them to air dry completely.

4. Prepare Your Skin

Always clean your skin thoroughly before applying DMSO. Residues from soaps, lotions, or deodorants can mix with the solution and enter your body. Follow the preparation steps outlined in **4.1** to ensure the area is contaminant-free.

5. Work in a Clean Environment

Set up a workspace that minimizes exposure to dust, oils, or debris. Use a silicone mat or clean cloth to protect your surfaces, and keep your workspace free from food, drinks, or other distractions.

Troubleshooting Contamination

Even with the best precautions, contamination can sometimes happen. Here's how to identify and address common issues:

- **Cloudy Solution**: If your DMSO appears cloudy, it may have absorbed moisture or contaminants. Discard and mix a fresh batch using distilled water.
- **Sticky Residue**: Sticky or tacky DMSO may indicate impurities. Clean your tools and surfaces, and start again with pure ingredients.
- **Skin Irritation**: If you notice redness or irritation after application, wash the area with cool water immediately and inspect your tools, skin preparation, and DMSO for potential contaminants.

Pro Tips for Maximum Purity

- **Distilled Water Only**: When diluting DMSO, use distilled water instead of tap water, which can contain minerals and impurities.
- **Label Everything**: Keep your solutions and tools clearly labeled to avoid mix-ups.
- **Store Smart**: Keep your DMSO and tools in a cool, dry place away from sunlight and heat, which can degrade the solution over time.

Why It Matters

Avoiding contaminants isn't just about keeping your DMSO solutions clean—it's about protecting your body and ensuring the compound can do its job effectively. By prioritizing purity at every step, you're maximizing the benefits of DMSO while minimizing risks. It's a small investment of effort with big rewards for your health.

As we continue, we'll explore how to manage sensitivities and reactions, giving you even more tools to use DMSO confidently and safely.

4.3 Managing Sensitivities and Reactions

For all its benefits, DMSO isn't without its quirks. Some users experience mild reactions when first using the compound, while others may notice sensitivities that need a little troubleshooting. The good news is that most of these issues are easily manageable with the right knowledge and preparation. Let's explore how to navigate sensitivities and ensure a smooth experience with DMSO.

Understanding Sensitivities

Reactions to DMSO are often a result of its unique properties. Because it penetrates the skin and carries substances into the body, your response can depend on several factors, including the concentration of DMSO, the condition of your skin, and even how your body processes sulfur compounds. Here are the most common reactions:

- **Mild Skin Irritation**: Redness, warmth, or a slight burning sensation may occur, especially with higher concentrations or sensitive skin.

- **Garlic-Like Odor**: A harmless but distinctive smell on your breath or skin, caused by DMSO's metabolism into dimethyl sulfide.
- **Temporary Dryness**: DMSO can pull water from the skin, leading to dryness or flakiness after use.

These reactions are typically mild and temporary, but understanding how to manage them is key to making the most of your DMSO experience.

How to Minimize Reactions

1. Start with a Lower Concentration

- For first-time users or those with sensitive skin, begin with a 30%–50% dilution. This allows your body to adjust to DMSO gradually.
- As your comfort level increases, you can experiment with higher concentrations for specific applications.

2. Patch Test Before Full Application

- Apply a small amount of diluted DMSO to a discreet area, like the inside of your wrist or forearm.
- Wait 24 hours to observe any reactions before proceeding with a larger application.

3. Keep Skin Clean and Dry

- Follow the preparation steps outlined in **4.1** to ensure the application area is free of residues or irritants that could interact with DMSO.

4. Moisturize After Use

- If you notice dryness or flaking, apply a fragrance-free, oil-free moisturizer after the DMSO has fully absorbed (20–30 minutes). Aloe vera gel is a great option for soothing and hydrating the skin.

Troubleshooting Common Reactions

Even with careful preparation, you might encounter occasional sensitivities. Here's how to handle them:

- **Redness or Warmth**: This is often a sign that the concentration is too high. Dilute your solution further and reapply.
- **Itchiness or Burning**: Wash the area with cool water immediately. If the sensation persists, discontinue use and consult a professional.
- **Persistent Odor**: The garlic-like smell is harmless but can be minimized by drinking plenty of water to support your body's natural detox processes.

When to Seek Professional Advice

While most reactions are minor and manageable, there are instances where professional guidance is recommended:

- **Severe Skin Irritation**: If redness, swelling, or discomfort persists after dilution and proper cleaning, consult a healthcare provider.
- **Unusual Symptoms**: Headaches, nausea, or other unexpected reactions may indicate an underlying sensitivity to sulfur compounds.

Tips for Long-Term Comfort

If you plan to use DMSO regularly, these strategies can help maintain comfort and prevent sensitivities over time:

- **Rotate Application Sites**: Avoid applying DMSO to the same area repeatedly to give your skin time to recover.
- **Stay Hydrated**: Drinking water supports your body's natural ability to process DMSO and minimize side effects.
- **Monitor Your Progress**: Keep a journal of your applications and any reactions to identify patterns and make adjustments.

A Personalized Approach

No two bodies are exactly alike, and your experience with DMSO may differ from someone else's. The key is to approach it with patience and curiosity, treating each reaction as an opportunity to learn what works best for you. With these strategies, you'll be well-equipped to manage sensitivities and unlock the full potential of DMSO safely and confidently.

4.4 Dos and Don'ts of DMSO Use

Using DMSO effectively and safely comes down to following a few key principles. While this versatile compound can be a game-changer for health and wellness, its powerful properties demand respect. To make it easy, here's a straightforward guide to the dos and don'ts of working with DMSO, complete with a table for quick reference.

Why Guidelines Matter

DMSO's ability to penetrate the skin and carry substances directly into the body is both its greatest strength and its biggest responsibility. Following the right practices ensures that you harness its benefits while avoiding unnecessary risks. Think of these dos and don'ts as your DMSO playbook.

Dos and Don'ts: At a Glance

Do	Don't
Use Pharmaceutical-Grade DMSO: Ensure you're working with 99.9% pure, high-quality DMSO to avoid contaminants.	**Use Industrial-Grade DMSO**: It may contain impurities or residues unsuitable for therapeutic use.
Dilute Appropriately: Adjust concentration based on the sensitivity of the application area (e.g., 30% for delicate skin).	**Apply Undiluted DMSO to Sensitive Skin**: High concentrations can cause irritation or burning.
Clean Skin Thoroughly: Wash the area with fragrance-free soap and water to remove residues or impurities.	**Skip Skin Preparation**: Dirt, oils, or lotions on the skin can mix with DMSO and enter the bloodstream.
Use Glass Tools and Containers: DMSO can leach chemicals from plastic, so stick to glass or stainless steel.	**Store or Mix DMSO in Plastic**: Plastics can degrade and contaminate the solution.
Apply with Clean Applicators: Use cotton balls, gauze, or natural fiber brushes, and discard after each use.	**Reuse Applicators**: Old applicators can introduce bacteria or impurities into your DMSO solution.

Work in a Clean, Ventilated Area: Minimize exposure to contaminants by keeping your workspace organized and free of distractions.	**Mix or Store DMSO in Dusty or Cluttered Areas:** Contaminants in the environment can compromise your solution.
Label and Store Properly: Use amber glass bottles, label dilutions clearly, and store in a cool, dry place.	**Expose DMSO to Sunlight or Heat:** Prolonged exposure can degrade the compound and reduce effectiveness.
Test on a Small Area First: Perform a patch test to check for sensitivities before widespread application.	**Skip the Patch Test:** Applying DMSO broadly without testing can lead to unexpected reactions.
Stay Hydrated: Drink plenty of water to support your body as it metabolizes DMSO.	**Neglect Hydration:** Dehydration can amplify side effects like dryness or odor.
Consult a Professional for Internal Use: Seek guidance before using DMSO internally to ensure safe and appropriate practices.	**Experiment with Internal Use Without Guidance:** Improper use can result in adverse effects.

Best Practices for Everyday Use

1. Start Low, Go Slow

If you're new to DMSO, begin with a lower concentration (e.g., 30%–50%) and increase gradually as needed. This helps your body adjust while minimizing the risk of irritation.

2. Keep It Simple

Avoid overcomplicating your routine. Stick to clean tools, simple solutions, and a consistent workspace to keep your process straightforward and effective.

3. Monitor Your Reactions

Pay attention to how your body responds. While mild redness or a garlic-like odor is normal, any persistent discomfort or unusual symptoms should prompt a reevaluation of your technique or concentration.

Why It's Worth the Effort

Following these dos and don'ts ensures that your DMSO experience is both safe and effective. By respecting its powerful properties and approaching it with care, you're setting yourself up for success while protecting your body from unnecessary risks.

As we move forward, you'll learn how to apply DMSO for specific conditions and harness its full potential with confidence.

Part III

REMEDIES BY CONDITION

Chapter 5

PAIN RELIEF

5.1 Remedies for Joint Pain and Arthritis

Joint pain can be a relentless companion. Whether it's the persistent ache of arthritis or the sharp sting of inflammation after a long day, it affects not only your mobility but your quality of life. I remember my first brush with chronic joint pain—it felt like my knees had aged decades overnight. The stiffness, the swelling, the frustration of not being able to move freely—it was exhausting. That's when I discovered DMSO.

DMSO, with its anti-inflammatory and pain-relieving properties, has been a game-changer. It doesn't just mask the pain—it works with your body to reduce swelling, improve circulation, and promote healing deep within the joints. Let's dive into the remedies that have made a difference for me and countless others.

Why DMSO Works for Joint Pain

Joint pain often stems from inflammation, restricted blood flow, or damage to the cartilage and tissues within the joint. DMSO addresses all three:

- **Anti-Inflammatory**: Reduces swelling and calms the immune response.
- **Analgesic**: Blocks pain signals for near-instant relief.
- **Deep Penetration**: Reaches tissues that most topical remedies can't, delivering healing directly where it's needed.

10+ Remedies for Joint Pain and Arthritis

1. General Joint Pain Relief Rub

- **What You'll Need:**
    - 70% DMSO solution
    - Cotton ball or gauze

- **How to Use:**
    - Clean the affected joint with mild soap and water.
    - Apply DMSO to the joint using a cotton ball or gauze.
    - Let it absorb for 20–30 minutes before rinsing with cool water.

- **Personal Note**: This was my first introduction to DMSO, and the immediate relief felt like a revelation.

2. Arthritis Hand Soak

- **What You'll Need:**
    - 50% DMSO solution
    - Warm water
    - Large bowl

- **How to Use:**
  - Mix 1 cup of DMSO with 4 cups of warm water in a bowl.
  - Soak your hands for 15–20 minutes.
  - Rinse with cool water and pat dry.
- **Benefits:** Loosens stiff joints and reduces swelling.
- **Personal Note:** My mother swears by this soak for her morning stiffness—it's now a part of her daily ritual.

3. Magnesium-Infused Joint Rub

- **What You'll Need:**
  - 70% DMSO solution
  - 1 teaspoon magnesium oil
- **How to Use:**
  - Mix DMSO with magnesium oil in a glass container.
  - Massage gently into the joint.
  - Let it absorb for 20–30 minutes before rinsing.
- **Benefits:** Combines DMSO's penetration with magnesium's muscle-relaxing properties.

4. Warm Compress for Deep Relief

- **What You'll Need:**
  - 50% DMSO solution
  - Warm, damp towel
- **How to Use:**
  - Apply DMSO to the joint with a cotton pad.
  - Cover with the warm towel for 15–20 minutes.
  - Remove the towel and let the area air dry.

- **Personal Note**: This is my go-to after a long hike—it feels like a spa treatment for sore knees.

5. Overnight Relief Wrap

- **What You'll Need:**
  - 70% DMSO solution
  - Soft cloth or gauze
  - Elastic bandage
- **How to Use:**
  - Soak the cloth in DMSO and wrap it around the joint.
  - Secure with an elastic bandage.
  - Leave it on overnight, then rinse in the morning.
- **Benefits**: Delivers sustained relief while you sleep.

6. DMSO and Turmeric Paste

- **What You'll Need:**
  - 50% DMSO solution
  - 1/2 teaspoon turmeric powder
  - 1 teaspoon distilled water
- **How to Use:**
  - Mix turmeric with water to form a paste.
  - Add DMSO and mix thoroughly.
  - Apply to the joint and leave for 15–20 minutes before rinsing.
- **Benefits**: Combines the anti-inflammatory properties of turmeric with DMSO's deep-tissue benefits.

7. Aloe Vera and DMSO Blend

- **What You'll Need:**
    - 50% DMSO solution
    - 1 tablespoon aloe vera gel
- **How to Use:**
    - Mix DMSO with aloe vera gel.
    - Apply a thin layer to the joint.
    - Allow it to absorb for 20–30 minutes before rinsing.
- **Benefits**: Soothes the skin while reducing joint inflammation.

8. Cooling Peppermint Gel

- **What You'll Need:**
    - 50% DMSO solution
    - 1 teaspoon aloe vera gel
    - 3 drops peppermint essential oil
- **How to Use:**
    - Mix the ingredients in a glass container.
    - Apply to the joint using clean hands or a cotton pad.
    - Let it absorb fully.
- **Personal Note**: This one is perfect for summer days—it cools and refreshes as it works.

9. Joint Recovery Bath

- **What You'll Need:**
    - 1/4 cup 50% DMSO solution
    - 1 cup Epsom salts
    - Warm water

- How to Use:
    - Add ingredients to a warm bath.
    - Soak for 20 minutes, focusing on submerging the affected joint.
    - Rinse with cool water afterward.
- **Benefits**: Perfect for whole-body relief when multiple joints are sore.

Tips for Success

- **Stay Active**: Gentle movement keeps joints flexible and supports recovery.
- **Be Consistent**: Regular application yields the best results for chronic pain.
- **Listen to Your Body**: Adjust concentrations and frequency based on your comfort level.

Freedom to Move

These remedies aren't just about managing pain—they're about reclaiming your ability to move freely and enjoy life. DMSO has been my partner in overcoming joint stiffness, and I hope these solutions help you find the same relief and empowerment.

Next, we'll tackle remedies for muscle soreness and tension, exploring more ways to support your body's recovery.

5.2 Solutions for Muscle Recovery and Tension Relief

Muscle soreness has a way of sneaking up on you, whether it's from an intense workout, a long day on your feet, or the creeping tension that builds after hours at a desk. I've been there—the dull ache, the tightness that makes every movement feel like a chore. The good news is, DMSO can offer relief that's not only effective but feels almost magical in its simplicity.

When I first started using DMSO for muscle soreness, I was skeptical. Could something so straightforward really work for deep-seated tension? But after a few applications, I became a believer. My post-workout recovery times shrank, and those lingering aches that seemed impervious to stretching and heat packs started to melt away. Let's dive into the remedies that helped me—and can help you too.

Why DMSO Works for Muscle Recovery

Muscle soreness often results from inflammation, microtears in muscle fibers, or lactic acid buildup. DMSO addresses all three. Its anti-inflammatory properties reduce swelling, its penetration capabilities allow it to target deep tissues, and its circulation-enhancing effects flush out toxins and lactic acid. Whether it's for a one-time strain or chronic tension, DMSO adapts to your body's needs.

10+ Effective Remedies for Muscle Soreness and Tension

1. Post-Workout Recovery Rub

- **What You'll Need:**
    - 70% DMSO solution
    - 1 teaspoon magnesium oil
    - 3 drops peppermint essential oil
- **How to Use:**
    - Mix the ingredients in a small glass container.
    - Massage into sore muscles using clean hands or a cotton pad.
    - Allow it to absorb for 20–30 minutes before rinsing.

- **Personal Note**: After an intense leg day, this rub became my go-to. The cooling effect of the peppermint felt like an instant reward for my hard work.

2. Cooling Peppermint Muscle Spray

- **What You'll Need:**
    - 50% DMSO solution
    - 1 tablespoon distilled water
    - 5 drops peppermint essential oil
- **How to Use:**
    - Combine the ingredients in a glass spray bottle.
    - Shake well and spritz directly onto sore muscles.
    - Massage gently for even application.
- **Frequency**: Use as needed.
- **Personal Note**: Perfect for those days when you just can't be bothered with creams. A quick spray and a gentle rub, and I'm good to go.

3. Warm Compress for Deep Relief

- **What You'll Need:**
    - 70% DMSO solution
    - Warm, damp towel
- **How to Use:**
    - Apply DMSO to the affected area using a clean applicator.
    - Cover the area with the warm towel for 15–20 minutes.
    - Let the area air dry naturally.
- **Benefits**: Relaxes tight muscles and enhances circulation.

- **Personal Note**: I use this whenever I've slept in an awkward position, and it's a lifesaver.

4. Lavender and Eucalyptus Soothing Gel

- **What You'll Need:**
    - 50% DMSO solution
    - 1 tablespoon aloe vera gel
    - 2 drops lavender essential oil
    - 2 drops eucalyptus essential oil
- **How to Use:**
    - Mix the ingredients in a glass container.
    - Apply a thin layer to the affected area.
    - Let it absorb for 20–30 minutes before rinsing.
- **Benefits**: Combines DMSO's muscle-relaxing properties with the calming effects of essential oils.

5. Muscle Recovery Bath Soak

- **What You'll Need:**
    - 1/4 cup DMSO (50% solution)
    - 1 cup Epsom salts
    - 5 drops lavender essential oil
- **How to Use:**
    - Add ingredients to a warm bath and mix well.
    - Soak for 20 minutes, ensuring the sore muscles are submerged.
    - Rinse with cool water after soaking.
- **Personal Note**: My ultimate treat after a long hike—pure relaxation in a tub.

6. Anti-Inflammatory Turmeric Blend

- **What You'll Need:**
  - 70% DMSO solution
  - 1/2 teaspoon turmeric powder
  - 1 teaspoon distilled water
- **How to Use:**
  - Mix the turmeric with water to form a paste.
  - Add the DMSO and mix thoroughly.
  - Apply to the sore area and leave for 15 minutes before rinsing.
- **Benefits**: Combines the anti-inflammatory effects of turmeric with DMSO's deep-tissue benefits.

7. Overnight Muscle Wrap

- **What You'll Need:**
  - 70% DMSO solution
  - Soft cloth or gauze
  - Elastic bandage
- **How to Use:**
  - Soak the cloth in DMSO and wrap it around the sore muscle.
  - Secure with an elastic bandage, ensuring it's snug but not tight.
  - Leave overnight and rinse in the morning.
- **Personal Note**: This wrap has been a game-changer for my shoulder tension.

8. Ginger and Magnesium Rub

- **What You'll Need:**
    - 50% DMSO solution
    - 1 teaspoon magnesium oil
    - 1/2 teaspoon grated ginger juice

- **How to Use:**
    - Mix the ingredients thoroughly.
    - Apply a thin layer to the affected area and massage gently.
    - Allow it to absorb for 20 minutes before rinsing.

- **Benefits**: Combines ginger's warming properties with magnesium's muscle-relaxing effects.

Tips for Better Recovery

- **Hydrate Well**: DMSO supports detoxification, so drinking water helps flush out toxins.
- **Stretch It Out**: Combine DMSO remedies with light stretching to enhance recovery.
- **Be Consistent**: Regular use yields the best results, especially for chronic soreness.

Relief Within Reach

These remedies aren't just about easing soreness—they're about empowering you to take control of your recovery. Whether you're recovering from a marathon or dealing with everyday muscle tension, DMSO can help you feel like yourself again. From quick sprays to soothing wraps, there's a remedy here for every situation.

Next, we'll explore solutions for managing chronic pain—a deeper challenge that DMSO is uniquely equipped to tackle.

5.3 Managing Chronic Pain: A Comprehensive Guide

Living with chronic pain is like carrying an invisible weight that no one else can see. It's not just the physical discomfort—it's the exhaustion, the frustration, and the search for something, anything, that works. I've walked that path, and I know how relentless it can feel. That's why I'm so passionate about DMSO. It's not a cure-all, but for many, it's a lifeline—a tool to take back control and find relief where other solutions have fallen short.

DMSO is uniquely suited for chronic pain because it doesn't just mask the symptoms; it addresses the inflammation, nerve irritation, and cellular damage at the root of the problem. Let's explore how this incredible compound can help you navigate chronic pain and improve your quality of life.

Why DMSO is Effective for Chronic Pain

Chronic pain often has multiple causes, from persistent inflammation to nerve damage or even poor circulation. DMSO's versatility makes it ideal for tackling these issues:

- **Reduces Inflammation**: Calms the overactive immune response that causes swelling and discomfort.
- **Blocks Pain Signals**: Acts as a natural analgesic, interrupting nerve conduction for near-instant relief.
- **Enhances Healing**: Improves circulation and cellular repair, addressing the underlying damage.

10+ Remedies for Chronic Pain

1. Full-Body Pain Relief Rub

- **What You'll Need:**
  - 70% DMSO solution
  - 1 tablespoon magnesium oil
  - 5 drops lavender essential oil
- **How to Use:**
  - Mix the ingredients in a glass container.
  - Massage into affected areas using clean hands or a cotton pad.
  - Let it absorb for 20–30 minutes before rinsing.
- **Benefits**: Provides widespread relief and promotes relaxation.
- **Personal Note**: This has become my nighttime ritual after long, physically demanding days.

2. Nerve Pain Cooling Spray

- **What You'll Need:**
  - 50% DMSO solution
  - 1 tablespoon distilled water
  - 3 drops peppermint essential oil
  - 2 drops eucalyptus essential oil
- **How to Use:**
  - Combine the ingredients in a glass spray bottle.
  - Shake well and spritz directly onto areas of nerve pain.
  - Massage gently for even application.
- **Benefits**: Soothes irritated nerves and reduces discomfort.

- **Personal Note**: A lifesaver for my sciatic nerve flare-ups—it provides almost instant relief.

3. Deep Tissue Warm Compress

- **What You'll Need:**
    - 70% DMSO solution
    - Warm, damp towel
- **How to Use:**
    - Apply DMSO to the affected area with a cotton pad.
    - Cover the area with the warm towel for 15–20 minutes.
    - Let the area air dry naturally.
- **Benefits**: Penetrates deep tissues for sustained relief.

4. Pain Management Bath Soak

- **What You'll Need:**
    - 1/4 cup 50% DMSO solution
    - 1 cup Epsom salts
    - 5 drops chamomile essential oil
- **How to Use:**
    - Add ingredients to a warm bath and mix well.
    - Soak for 20 minutes, focusing on submerging areas of chronic pain.
    - Rinse with cool water afterward.
- **Benefits**: Combines the soothing effects of Epsom salts and chamomile with DMSO's deep-tissue action.

5. Turmeric and DMSO Paste

- **What You'll Need:**
    - 50% DMSO solution
    - 1 teaspoon turmeric powder
    - 1 teaspoon distilled water

- **How to Use:**
    - Mix turmeric with water to form a paste.
    - Add DMSO and mix thoroughly.
    - Apply to the affected area and leave for 15–20 minutes before rinsing.

- **Benefits**: Targets inflammation and supports joint and tissue recovery.

6. Chronic Pain Daily Spray

- **What You'll Need:**
    - 50% DMSO solution
    - 1 tablespoon distilled water
    - 3 drops frankincense essential oil

- **How to Use:**
    - Mix ingredients in a glass spray bottle.
    - Spritz onto affected areas twice daily.
    - Massage gently for even coverage.

- **Benefits**: Easy-to-apply, portable solution for ongoing pain relief.

7. Stress-Relieving Lavender Wrap

- **What You'll Need:**
    - 70% DMSO solution
    - Soft cloth or gauze
    - Elastic bandage
    - 2 drops lavender essential oil
- **How to Use:**
    - Add lavender oil to the DMSO solution and soak the cloth.
    - Wrap it around the painful area and secure with the elastic bandage.
    - Leave on for 1–2 hours before removing and rinsing.
- **Benefits**: Combines DMSO's pain relief with lavender's calming properties.

8. Anti-Inflammatory Vitamin C Blend

- **What You'll Need:**
    - 50% DMSO solution
    - 1/4 teaspoon powdered vitamin C
    - 1 teaspoon distilled water
- **How to Use:**
    - Mix vitamin C with water until dissolved.
    - Add DMSO and stir gently.
    - Apply to the affected area and let it absorb for 20 minutes.
- **Benefits**: Enhances collagen repair and reduces inflammation.

Tips for Chronic Pain Management

- **Be Consistent**: Regular use is key to managing long-term pain.
- **Combine Therapies**: Pair DMSO remedies with other approaches like stretching, acupuncture, or physical therapy.
- **Track Your Progress**: Keep a journal of applications and results to identify what works best for you.

Finding Relief, One Step at a Time

Chronic pain doesn't have to define your life. With DMSO, you have a tool that addresses the root causes of discomfort while offering meaningful relief. These remedies aren't just solutions—they're small acts of reclaiming your freedom and rediscovering what it feels like to move, rest, and live without constant pain.

CHAPTER 6

SKIN HEALTH AND WOUND HEALING

6.1 Managing Chronic Skin Conditions

Living with chronic skin conditions can feel like a never-ending battle. Whether it's the persistent irritation of eczema, the stubborn plaques of psoriasis, or the relentless discomfort of chronic itching, these conditions often take a toll far beyond the surface. I've seen firsthand how these challenges affect not just your skin, but your confidence and peace of mind. That's where DMSO comes in—a natural, powerful ally that works with your body to soothe, heal, and restore balance.

Why DMSO Works for Chronic Skin Conditions

Chronic skin conditions often stem from inflammation, immune dysfunction, or disruptions in the skin's protective barrier. DMSO tackles these root causes with its unique properties:

- **Anti-Inflammatory**: Reduces redness, swelling, and irritation by calming overactive immune responses.
- **Cellular Repair**: Promotes healing by increasing blood flow and oxygen delivery to damaged tissues.
- **Hydration and Barrier Support**: Improves moisture retention and strengthens the skin's natural barrier when combined with complementary agents like aloe vera.

10+ Remedies for Chronic Skin Conditions

1. Soothing Eczema Relief Gel

- **What You'll Need:**
  - 50% DMSO solution
  - 1 tablespoon aloe vera gel
  - 3 drops chamomile essential oil

- **How to Use:**
  - Mix the ingredients in a glass container.
  - Apply a thin layer to affected areas using clean hands or a cotton pad.
  - Let it absorb for 20–30 minutes before rinsing.

- **Benefits**: Reduces redness and hydrates dry, flaky skin.
- **Personal Note**: This blend was a game-changer for my friend's eczema—it's now her go-to remedy.

2. Psoriasis Flare-Up Spray

- **What You'll Need:**
  - 50% DMSO solution
  - 1 tablespoon distilled water

- o 3 drops tea tree oil
- o 2 drops lavender essential oil

- **How to Use:**
  - o Combine the ingredients in a glass spray bottle.
  - o Shake well and spritz onto affected areas.
  - o Let it air dry; no need to rinse.

- **Frequency**: Use twice daily during flare-ups.
- **Benefits**: Soothes inflammation and reduces plaque formation.

3. Anti-Itch Calming Rub

- **What You'll Need:**
  - o 70% DMSO solution
  - o 1 teaspoon magnesium oil
  - o 2 drops peppermint essential oil

- **How to Use:**
  - o Mix the ingredients in a glass container.
  - o Massage gently into itchy areas using clean hands or a cotton pad.
  - o Allow it to absorb fully; rinse if irritation persists.

- **Personal Note**: A lifesaver during allergy season when my skin felt like it was on fire.

4. Chronic Skin Soothing Wrap

- **What You'll Need:**
  - o 70% DMSO solution
  - o Soft cloth or gauze
  - o Elastic bandage

- **How to Use:**
  - Soak the cloth in DMSO and wrap it around the irritated area.
  - Secure with an elastic bandage and leave on for 1–2 hours.
  - Remove the wrap and rinse with cool water.
- **Benefits**: Provides deep, sustained relief for persistent discomfort.

5. Vitamin E and DMSO Serum

- **What You'll Need:**
  - 50% DMSO solution
  - 1 capsule of vitamin E oil
- **How to Use:**
  - Puncture the vitamin E capsule and mix the oil with the DMSO.
  - Apply to affected areas using clean hands.
  - Let it absorb for 20 minutes before rinsing.
- **Benefits**: Repairs the skin barrier and reduces scarring.

6. Aloe and Calendula Healing Gel

- **What You'll Need:**
  - 50% DMSO solution
  - 1 tablespoon aloe vera gel
  - 2 drops calendula oil
- **How to Use:**
  - Mix the ingredients in a glass container.
  - Apply a thin layer to irritated areas and let it absorb.
  - Rinse after 30 minutes if needed.
- **Personal Note**: A gentle, effective remedy for soothing flare-ups and reducing redness.

Tips for Chronic Skin Management

- **Patch Test First**: Always test a small area before applying DMSO to large sections of skin.
- **Hydrate Regularly**: Drink plenty of water to support overall skin health and aid recovery.
- **Be Consistent**: Chronic conditions respond best to regular, ongoing treatment.

A Path to Comfort

Chronic skin conditions can feel overwhelming, but DMSO offers a way to take control and find relief. These remedies are more than just solutions—they're steps toward reclaiming your confidence and comfort. Whether you're managing eczema, psoriasis, or persistent itchiness, DMSO provides a natural, effective way to support your skin's healing journey.

In the next section, we'll explore remedies for renewing and repairing the skin, including solutions for scars, stretch marks, and anti-aging.

6.2 Skin Renewal and Repair

Skin tells a story—of growth, experiences, and even the challenges we've faced. But sometimes, scars, stretch marks, and signs of aging can feel like chapters we'd rather rewrite. Whether it's the aftermath of an injury, the lingering stretch marks from a life-changing pregnancy, or the fine lines that whisper of time's passing, DMSO offers a way to renew and repair. Its unique ability to penetrate deep into the skin and support cellular regeneration makes it a powerful ally in reclaiming your skin's natural beauty.

Why DMSO Works for Skin Renewal

DMSO doesn't just work on the surface; it gets to the root of the problem. By increasing blood flow, delivering nutrients, and supporting collagen production, it addresses the underlying causes of scars, stretch marks, and wrinkles. Combined with complementary agents like aloe vera, vitamin E, or essential oils, it becomes even more effective.

10+ Remedies for Skin Renewal and Repair

1. Scar-Soothing Vitamin E Serum

- **What You'll Need:**
    - 50% DMSO solution
    - 1 capsule of vitamin E oil
- **How to Use:**
    - Mix the vitamin E oil with the DMSO in a small glass container.
    - Apply a thin layer to the scarred area using clean fingers.
    - Let it absorb for 20–30 minutes before rinsing.
- **Benefits**: Helps fade scars and softens tissue over time.
- **Personal Note**: I used this on a burn scar, and over a few weeks, the difference was astonishing.

2. Stretch Mark Reduction Gel

- **What You'll Need:**
    - 50% DMSO solution
    - 1 tablespoon aloe vera gel
    - 2 drops rosehip oil

- **How to Use:**
  - Combine the ingredients in a glass container.
  - Massage into stretch marks using circular motions.
  - Allow it to absorb fully; no rinsing needed.
- **Benefits**: Improves elasticity and reduces discoloration.

3. Collagen-Boosting DMSO Blend

- **What You'll Need:**
  - 50% DMSO solution
  - 1 teaspoon collagen powder
  - 1 teaspoon distilled water
- **How to Use:**
  - Dissolve the collagen powder in water.
  - Mix with the DMSO and apply to the targeted area.
  - Let it sit for 20 minutes before rinsing.
- **Benefits**: Supports skin elasticity and firmness.

4. Anti-Aging Night Serum

- **What You'll Need:**
  - 50% DMSO solution
  - 1 teaspoon aloe vera gel
  - 3 drops frankincense essential oil
- **How to Use:**
  - Combine ingredients in a glass dropper bottle.
  - Apply a thin layer to the face and neck before bedtime.
  - Leave overnight and rinse in the morning.

- **Benefits**: Reduces fine lines and hydrates the skin.
- **Personal Note**: I've incorporated this into my nightly routine, and my skin feels smoother and more hydrated.

5. Green Tea and DMSO Scar Treatment

- **What You'll Need:**
    - 50% DMSO solution
    - 1 teaspoon brewed green tea (cooled)
- **How to Use:**
    - Mix the green tea with DMSO in a small container.
    - Apply to the scarred area using a cotton pad.
    - Let it absorb for 15–20 minutes before rinsing.
- **Benefits**: Combines the antioxidant power of green tea with DMSO's deep-tissue repair.

6. Cocoa Butter Stretch Mark Balm

- **What You'll Need:**
    - 50% DMSO solution
    - 1 tablespoon cocoa butter
- **How to Use:**
    - Warm the cocoa butter slightly to soften it.
    - Mix with the DMSO and apply to stretch marks.
    - Massage thoroughly and leave overnight.
- **Benefits**: Hydrates and improves skin texture.

7. Overnight Skin Rejuvenation Wrap

- **What You'll Need:**
    - 70% DMSO solution
    - Soft gauze or cloth
    - Elastic bandage
- **How to Use:**
    - Soak the gauze in DMSO and wrap it around the targeted area (e.g., arms or thighs).
    - Secure with the bandage and leave on overnight.
    - Remove in the morning and rinse with cool water.
- **Benefits**: Supports deep-tissue repair and hydration during sleep.

Tips for Skin Renewal

- **Be Patient**: Scars and stretch marks take time to fade. Regular use of DMSO remedies accelerates the process but requires consistency.
- **Hydrate Your Skin**: Pair DMSO with hydrating agents like aloe vera or cocoa butter to prevent dryness.
- **Protect from Sunlight**: Use sunscreen on treated areas during the day, as healing skin can be more sensitive to UV rays.

A New Chapter for Your Skin

DMSO doesn't erase history, but it helps you rewrite the parts of your story etched into your skin. These remedies provide a practical, empowering way to reduce scars, fade stretch marks, and restore a youthful glow. With time, patience, and consistency, your skin can feel as vibrant and confident as you are.

Next, we'll tackle remedies for treating acute skin issues, including acne spots, burns, and wound healing.

6.3 Treating Acute Skin Issues

Acne, burns, and wounds are among the most frustrating skin challenges. Whether it's the stubborn blemish that appears right before an important event, the sting of a burn, or the slow healing of a cut, these issues demand attention—and fast. DMSO offers a powerful, natural solution for treating these acute skin issues, working deep within the skin to promote rapid healing, reduce inflammation, and minimize scarring.

When I first discovered DMSO's potential for skin repair, I was skeptical. But after using it on a particularly nasty burn, I was amazed at how quickly the pain subsided and how minimal the scar was afterward. That experience made me a lifelong advocate. Let's explore how you can harness DMSO to address your skin's urgent needs.

Why DMSO Works for Acute Skin Issues

Acute skin issues often involve a mix of inflammation, microbial presence, and tissue damage. DMSO tackles these problems simultaneously:

- **Anti-Inflammatory**: Reduces redness, swelling, and discomfort.
- **Antimicrobial**: Inhibits the growth of bacteria and fungi, reducing infection risks.
- **Cellular Repair**: Enhances blood flow and oxygen delivery to promote faster healing.

10+ Remedies for Treating Acute Skin Issues

1. Acne Spot Treatment

- **What You'll Need:**
  - 50% DMSO solution
  - Cotton swab
- **How to Use:**
  - Dip the cotton swab in the DMSO solution.
  - Apply directly to blemishes, avoiding the surrounding skin.
  - Let it absorb for 10–15 minutes before rinsing.
- **Benefits**: Reduces redness and inflammation while speeding up healing.
- **Personal Note**: This became my emergency go-to for surprise breakouts before big meetings or events.

2. Antibacterial Wound Spray

- **What You'll Need:**
  - 50% DMSO solution
  - 1 tablespoon distilled water
  - 3 drops tea tree essential oil
- **How to Use:**
  - Mix the ingredients in a glass spray bottle.
  - Shake well and spray directly onto cuts or abrasions.
  - Let it air dry; no rinsing needed.
- **Benefits**: Cleanses wounds and reduces the risk of infection.

3. Burn Relief Gel

- **What You'll Need:**
    - 50% DMSO solution
    - 1 tablespoon aloe vera gel
    - 2 drops lavender essential oil
- **How to Use:**
    - Mix the ingredients in a glass container.
    - Apply a thin layer to the burned area using clean hands.
    - Reapply as needed for ongoing relief.
- **Benefits**: Soothes pain, reduces redness, and prevents blistering.
- **Personal Note**: This remedy saved me after an unfortunate run-in with a hot pan.

4. Quick-Healing Scar Treatment

- **What You'll Need:**
    - 50% DMSO solution
    - 1 teaspoon vitamin E oil
- **How to Use:**
    - Mix the DMSO with vitamin E oil in a small container.
    - Apply to the healing wound once the skin has closed.
    - Use twice daily to minimize scarring.
- **Benefits**: Supports tissue repair and reduces discoloration.

5. Chronic Acne Soothing Mask

- **What You'll Need:**
    - 50% DMSO solution
    - 1 teaspoon green tea extract
    - 1 teaspoon aloe vera gel

- **How to Use:**
  - Mix the ingredients into a smooth paste.
  - Apply to the affected areas and leave on for 15–20 minutes.
  - Rinse with cool water and pat dry.
- **Benefits**: Combines antioxidant protection with DMSO's deep-healing properties.

6. Wound Healing Compress

- **What You'll Need:**
  - 70% DMSO solution
  - Soft gauze or cloth
- **How to Use:**
  - Soak the gauze in DMSO and apply it to the wound (ensure the skin is closed).
  - Leave on for 30 minutes, then remove and rinse the area.
- **Benefits**: Speeds up healing and reduces inflammation.

7. Overnight Acne Spot Wrap

- **What You'll Need:**
  - 50% DMSO solution
  - Small piece of gauze
- **How to Use:**
  - Soak the gauze in DMSO and place it over the blemish.
  - Secure it with a bandage and leave it on overnight.
  - Remove and rinse in the morning.
- **Benefits**: Targets stubborn spots for faster resolution.

8. Cooling Lavender Burn Mist

- **What You'll Need:**
    - 50% DMSO solution
    - 1 tablespoon distilled water
    - 3 drops lavender essential oil
- **How to Use:**
    - Combine ingredients in a glass spray bottle.
    - Spray lightly over the burned area.
    - Reapply every 2–3 hours as needed.
- **Benefits**: Calms and hydrates damaged skin.

Tips for Treating Acute Skin Issues

- **Be Gentle**: Avoid rubbing or scrubbing damaged skin; let DMSO do the work.
- **Watch for Reactions**: Patch test on healthy skin before using on sensitive areas.
- **Stay Consistent**: Regular application yields the best results for faster healing.

Fast Relief, Long-Term Healing

Acute skin issues don't have to derail your day or leave lasting scars. With DMSO, you have a powerful tool to calm inflammation, promote healing, and restore your skin's natural health. These remedies aren't just quick fixes—they're solutions that empower you to take charge of your skin's recovery.

In the next chapter, we'll explore how DMSO can support digestive health and detoxification, taking its healing potential even further.

Chapter 7

RESPIRATORY AND IMMUNE SUPPORT

7.1 Sinus Infections and Congestion: Steam and Rinse Remedies

Few things disrupt daily life like congestion, sinus pressure, or breathing difficulties. Whether it's the lingering effects of a cold, chronic sinusitis, or even seasonal allergies, these issues make it hard to focus, rest, or feel like yourself. I've personally experienced the frustration of clogged sinuses that just won't clear and the exhaustion of shallow breathing during allergy season. DMSO has been a revelation for addressing these challenges, offering both immediate relief and long-term support for respiratory health.

Why DMSO Works for Lung and Sinus Relief

The respiratory system is highly sensitive to inflammation, irritants, and mucus buildup. DMSO offers multiple benefits:

- **Anti-Inflammatory**: Reduces swelling in nasal passages and airways.
- **Mucolytic**: Breaks down mucus, making it easier to expel.
- **Antimicrobial**: Inhibits the growth of bacteria and viruses that contribute to respiratory issues.

Its ability to penetrate tissues and work at a cellular level makes it uniquely suited for addressing respiratory problems.

10+ Remedies for Lung and Sinus Relief

1. Steam Inhalation for Sinus Congestion

- **What You'll Need:**
  - 1 teaspoon 50% DMSO solution
  - 4 cups boiling water
  - 3 drops eucalyptus essential oil
- **How to Use:**
  - Pour the boiling water into a large bowl and add DMSO and eucalyptus oil.
  - Lean over the bowl, covering your head with a towel to trap the steam.
  - Inhale deeply for 10–15 minutes.
- **Benefits**: Clears nasal passages and reduces sinus pressure.

- **Personal Note**: I swear by this remedy during allergy season—it's like hitting the reset button on my sinuses.

2. Chest Rub for Lung Inflammation

- **What You'll Need:**
    - 50% DMSO solution
    - 1 teaspoon coconut oil
    - 3 drops peppermint essential oil
- **How to Use:**
    - Mix the ingredients in a small container.
    - Massage onto your chest and upper back.
    - Cover with a warm towel for enhanced absorption.
- **Benefits**: Relieves chest tightness and promotes easier breathing.

3. Nasal Spray for Sinus Relief

- **What You'll Need:**
    - 10% DMSO solution
    - 1/4 teaspoon non-iodized sea salt
    - 1/2 cup distilled water
- **How to Use:**
    - Mix the ingredients in a sterile nasal spray bottle.
    - Spray 1–2 times in each nostril as needed.
- **Benefits**: Reduces inflammation and clears mucus buildup.
- **Personal Note**: This spray has become a staple during cold and flu season—simple but effective.

4. Ginger and DMSO Steam for Deep Lung Relief

- **What You'll Need:**
    - 1 teaspoon 50% DMSO solution
    - 4 cups boiling water
    - 1 teaspoon grated ginger
- **How to Use:**
    - Add grated ginger and DMSO to the boiling water.
    - Lean over the bowl and inhale the steam for 10 minutes.
- **Benefits**: Combines the anti-inflammatory properties of DMSO with ginger's soothing effects.

5. Overnight Chest Wrap

- **What You'll Need:**
    - 50% DMSO solution
    - Soft cloth or gauze
    - Elastic bandage
- **How to Use:**
    - Soak the cloth in DMSO and place it over your chest.
    - Secure with the elastic bandage and leave overnight.
    - Remove in the morning and rinse the area.
- **Benefits**: Provides sustained relief for chronic respiratory conditions.

6. Anti-Allergy Nasal Rinse

- **What You'll Need:**
    - 10% DMSO solution
    - 1/4 teaspoon baking soda
    - 1 cup distilled water

- **How to Use:**
  - Mix the ingredients in a sterile container.
  - Use a neti pot or nasal syringe to rinse each nostril.
  - Repeat once daily during allergy season.
- **Benefits**: Soothes irritation and removes allergens.

7. Peppermint and DMSO Lung Mist

- **What You'll Need:**
  - 50% DMSO solution
  - 1 tablespoon distilled water
  - 2 drops peppermint essential oil
- **How to Use:**
  - Combine ingredients in a glass spray bottle.
  - Spray lightly over your chest and upper back.
  - Massage gently for even absorption.
- **Benefits**: Clears airways and promotes deeper breathing.

8. Recovery Pack for Bronchitis

- **What You'll Need:**
  - 70% DMSO solution
  - Soft cloth
  - Elastic bandage
- **How to Use:**
  - Soak the cloth in DMSO and wrap it around your chest.
  - Secure with the elastic bandage and leave on for 1–2 hours.
  - Remove and rinse the area.
- **Benefits**: Reduces inflammation and supports recovery from bronchitis.

Tips for Respiratory Health

- **Stay Hydrated**: Drink plenty of water to help thin mucus and support respiratory function.
- **Combine with Lifestyle Adjustments**: Pair DMSO remedies with steam therapy, humidifiers, or allergen avoidance for better results.
- **Patch Test First**: Always test new solutions on a small area before widespread use, especially near sensitive areas like the nose.

Breathe Easy with DMSO

DMSO offers more than temporary relief—it supports your body's natural ability to heal and maintain clear, healthy airways. These remedies aren't just about fixing symptoms—they're about restoring your comfort and quality of life. Whether you're battling seasonal congestion or managing a chronic respiratory condition, DMSO is a powerful tool for finding relief.

In the next section, we'll explore how DMSO can boost immunity and enhance overall health, taking its benefits to the next level.

7.2 Chronic Respiratory Conditions: Asthma and Bronchitis Relief

Your immune system is your body's first line of defense, working tirelessly to fend off infections, repair damage, and maintain balance. But what happens when it needs a little extra support? Whether it's during cold and flu season, recovery from illness, or periods of high stress, DMSO can be a powerful ally for boosting your immune health. With its anti-inflammatory, antioxidant, and cellular-transport properties, DMSO enhances your body's natural defenses in ways few other remedies can.

When I first started using DMSO for immune support, it was during a particularly harsh winter. Between work stress and back-to-back colds, my body was drained. Incorporating DMSO into my wellness routine made a noticeable difference—it wasn't just about avoiding illness but feeling stronger and more resilient overall.

Why DMSO Supports Immune Health

DMSO's effects on the immune system are rooted in its unique abilities:

- **Anti-Inflammatory**: Reduces systemic inflammation, a common barrier to optimal immune function.
- **Antioxidant**: Scavenges free radicals, protecting immune cells from oxidative stress.
- **Carrier Molecule**: Enhances the delivery of immune-boosting agents, such as vitamin C or zinc, to the cells that need them most.

By addressing inflammation and supporting cellular repair, DMSO helps create an environment where the immune system can thrive.

10+ Remedies for Immune Support

1. General Immune Booster Spray

- **What You'll Need:**
    - 50% DMSO solution
    - 1 tablespoon distilled water
    - 3 drops frankincense essential oil
- **How to Use:**
    - Combine the ingredients in a glass spray bottle.

- - Shake well and spritz onto your chest or upper back.
  - Massage gently for even absorption.
- **Benefits**: Enhances immune response and supports respiratory health.

2. Vitamin C and DMSO Blend

- **What You'll Need:**
  - 50% DMSO solution
  - 1/4 teaspoon powdered vitamin C
  - 1 teaspoon distilled water
- **How to Use:**
  - Dissolve the vitamin C in water and mix with DMSO.
  - Apply to the wrists or inner forearms for systemic absorption.
  - Let it absorb for 20 minutes before rinsing.
- **Benefits**: Boosts immune function and fights oxidative stress.
- **Personal Note**: This blend became my go-to when I felt a cold coming on—it stopped it in its tracks more than once.

3. Antioxidant Detox Drink

- **What You'll Need:**
  - 1/4 teaspoon food-grade DMSO (diluted to 10%)
  - 1 cup water
  - Juice of 1/2 lemon
- **How to Use:**
  - Mix all ingredients in a glass container.
  - Drink slowly, preferably on an empty stomach.
- **Benefits**: Supports detoxification and boosts overall immune resilience.

4. Zinc-Infused Recovery Spray

- **What You'll Need:**
  - 50% DMSO solution
  - 1/4 teaspoon zinc sulfate powder
  - 1 tablespoon distilled water
- **How to Use:**
  - Dissolve the zinc sulfate in water and mix with DMSO.
  - Spray onto your chest or upper back.
  - Let it absorb for 20 minutes.
- **Benefits**: Combines DMSO's carrier properties with zinc's immune-strengthening effects.

5. Ginger and DMSO Immune Tea

- **What You'll Need:**
  - 1/4 teaspoon food-grade DMSO (diluted to 10%)
  - 1 cup hot water
  - 1 teaspoon grated ginger
- **How to Use:**
  - Steep the ginger in hot water for 5 minutes.
  - Add the DMSO once the tea has cooled slightly.
  - Sip slowly to support your immune system.
- **Benefits**: Combines the warming, anti-inflammatory properties of ginger with DMSO's detoxifying effects.

6. Recovery Wrap for Illness

- **What You'll Need:**
  - 50% DMSO solution
  - Soft cloth or gauze
  - Elastic bandage

- **How to Use:**
  - Soak the cloth in DMSO and wrap it around your wrists or ankles.
  - Secure with an elastic bandage and leave on for 1–2 hours.
  - Remove and rinse the area with cool water.

- **Benefits**: Provides systemic immune support during recovery.

7. Eucalyptus Steam for Immune Activation

- **What You'll Need:**
  - 1 teaspoon 50% DMSO solution
  - 4 cups boiling water
  - 3 drops eucalyptus essential oil

- **How to Use:**
  - Add the ingredients to a large bowl.
  - Lean over the bowl, covering your head with a towel, and inhale deeply for 10 minutes.

- **Benefits**: Clears respiratory pathways and supports immune defenses.

8. Lemon and DMSO Detox Drink

- **What You'll Need:**
  - 1/4 teaspoon food-grade DMSO (diluted to 10%)

- 1 cup warm water
- Juice of 1/2 lemon

- **How to Use:**
  - Mix ingredients and drink slowly in the morning.
  - Follow with a glass of plain water.

- **Benefits**: Detoxifies the body and boosts immune resilience.

Tips for Immune Support

- **Consistency is Key**: Regular use of DMSO remedies ensures lasting immune benefits.
- **Pair with Lifestyle Adjustments**: Eat nutrient-rich foods, stay active, and manage stress to complement DMSO's effects.
- **Listen to Your Body**: Adjust concentrations and methods based on your needs and sensitivities.

Strengthen Your Defenses

DMSO offers more than just symptom relief—it empowers your immune system to function at its best. These remedies provide practical, accessible ways to enhance your body's natural defenses, helping you stay healthy and resilient in the face of life's challenges.

In the next section, we'll explore how DMSO can support chronic respiratory conditions, offering targeted solutions for long-term relief.

7.3 Immune-Boosting Applications with DMSO

Living with chronic respiratory conditions like asthma, COPD, or persistent bronchitis can feel like a constant uphill battle. Breathing, something so fundamental, becomes a source of frustration and fatigue. I've watched loved ones struggle with these challenges, searching for ways to manage their symptoms and improve their quality of life. That's where DMSO can step in, offering a natural, multi-faceted approach to easing inflammation, clearing airways, and supporting lung health.

Why DMSO is Effective for Chronic Respiratory Health

Chronic respiratory conditions often involve ongoing inflammation, mucus buildup, and reduced oxygen exchange. DMSO's properties make it uniquely suited to address these issues:

- **Anti-Inflammatory**: Reduces swelling in airways, improving airflow.
- **Mucolytic**: Breaks down mucus, making it easier to expel.
- **Cellular Repair**: Promotes tissue healing and oxygen exchange, supporting long-term lung function.

When combined with complementary therapies, DMSO can make breathing easier and reduce the frequency and severity of flare-ups.

10+ Remedies for Chronic Respiratory Conditions

1. Steam Inhalation for Asthma Relief

- **What You'll Need:**
    - 1 teaspoon 50% DMSO solution
    - 4 cups boiling water
    - 3 drops eucalyptus essential oil

- **How to Use:**
  - Add the DMSO and eucalyptus oil to the boiling water in a large bowl.
  - Cover your head with a towel and inhale deeply for 10–15 minutes.
- **Benefits**: Reduces airway inflammation and clears mucus.
- **Personal Note**: This simple remedy has provided immediate relief for my partner's asthma during flare-ups.

2. Chest Rub for Persistent Coughs

- **What You'll Need:**
  - 50% DMSO solution
  - 1 teaspoon coconut oil
  - 3 drops peppermint essential oil
- **How to Use:**
  - Mix the ingredients in a small container.
  - Massage onto the chest and upper back.
  - Cover with a warm towel for enhanced absorption.
- **Benefits**: Soothes irritated airways and promotes deeper breathing.

3. Anti-Inflammatory Tea for Chronic Bronchitis

- **What You'll Need:**
  - 1/4 teaspoon food-grade DMSO (diluted to 10%)
  - 1 cup hot water
  - 1 teaspoon grated ginger
  - Juice of 1/2 lemon

- **How to Use:**
  - Steep the ginger in hot water for 5 minutes.
  - Add lemon juice and DMSO once the tea has cooled slightly.
  - Sip slowly, allowing the warm liquid to soothe your airways.
- **Benefits**: Combines the anti-inflammatory effects of ginger with DMSO's healing properties.

4. Overnight Lung Relief Pack

- **What You'll Need:**
  - 50% DMSO solution
  - Soft gauze or cloth
  - Elastic bandage
- **How to Use:**
  - Soak the gauze in DMSO and place it over your chest.
  - Secure with an elastic bandage and leave on overnight.
  - Remove in the morning and rinse the area.
- **Benefits**: Provides sustained relief for chronic conditions like COPD.

5. Mucus-Clearing Nasal Spray

- **What You'll Need:**
  - 10% DMSO solution
  - 1/4 teaspoon non-iodized sea salt
  - 1/2 cup distilled water
- **How to Use:**
  - Mix the ingredients in a sterile nasal spray bottle.
  - Spray 1–2 times in each nostril as needed.
- **Benefits**: Clears nasal passages and reduces mucus buildup.

6. Peppermint and Ginger Lung Mist

- **What You'll Need:**
    - 50% DMSO solution
    - 1 tablespoon distilled water
    - 2 drops peppermint essential oil
    - 1/2 teaspoon grated ginger juice

- **How to Use:**
    - Combine ingredients in a glass spray bottle.
    - Spray lightly over your chest and upper back.
    - Massage gently for even absorption.

- **Benefits**: Opens airways and soothes inflammation.

7. Anti-Allergy Foot Soak

- **What You'll Need:**
    - 1/4 cup 50% DMSO solution
    - Warm water (enough to fill a basin)
    - 1 teaspoon baking soda

- **How to Use:**
    - Add the ingredients to a basin of warm water.
    - Soak your feet for 20 minutes while relaxing.
    - Rinse and pat dry.

- **Benefits**: Supports detoxification and reduces systemic inflammation.

8. Turmeric and DMSO COPD Wrap

- **What You'll Need:**
    - 50% DMSO solution
    - 1/2 teaspoon turmeric powder
    - Soft gauze or cloth

- **How to Use:**
  - Mix the turmeric with the DMSO and soak the gauze in the solution.
  - Wrap the gauze around your chest and secure it with an elastic bandage.
  - Leave on for 1–2 hours before removing.
- **Benefits**: Combines turmeric's anti-inflammatory effects with DMSO's deep-tissue penetration.

Tips for Long-Term Respiratory Health

- **Stay Consistent**: Regular use of DMSO remedies helps manage chronic conditions over time.
- **Combine with Lifestyle Changes**: Avoid smoking, maintain a clean home environment, and use a humidifier to support lung health.
- **Monitor Symptoms**: Keep track of your progress and adjust remedies as needed.

Breathing Easier with DMSO

Chronic respiratory conditions may be long-term companions, but they don't have to define your life. DMSO offers practical, effective solutions for managing symptoms, reducing inflammation, and improving your overall quality of life. These remedies are designed to help you breathe easier—both literally and figuratively.

In the next chapter, we'll explore how DMSO supports digestive health and detoxification, expanding its role as a holistic healing tool.

Chapter 8

DIGESTIVE AND DETOXIFICATION REMEDIES

8.1 Gut Health: Remedies for IBS, SIBO, and Constipation

The gut is often called the body's second brain, and for good reason—it's central to overall health and well-being. But when something goes wrong, whether it's the unpredictable discomfort of IBS, the bloating of SIBO, or the frustration of constipation, it can throw your entire system off balance. I've experienced my fair share of digestive woes, from the occasional bloated evening to weeks of wondering why nothing seems to move right. It's these moments that made me turn to DMSO, and what a difference it has made.

With its anti-inflammatory properties, ability to transport nutrients, and role in cellular repair, DMSO offers unique support for gut health. Let's explore how this multitasking molecule can bring relief to even the most stubborn digestive issues.

Why DMSO Works for Gut Health

Digestive problems often stem from inflammation, microbial imbalances, or disruptions in the gut lining. DMSO addresses these root causes in several ways:

- **Anti-Inflammatory**: Reduces irritation and inflammation in the gut lining.
- **Antimicrobial**: Inhibits harmful bacteria, supporting a balanced microbiome.
- **Gut Barrier Repair**: Enhances tissue healing, strengthening the intestinal lining.

10+ Remedies for Digestive Health

1. Anti-Bloating Digestive Rub

- **What You'll Need:**
    - 50% DMSO solution
    - 1 teaspoon magnesium oil
    - 2 drops peppermint essential oil
- **How to Use:**
    - Mix the ingredients in a small container.
    - Massage onto the abdomen in circular motions.
    - Let it absorb for 20–30 minutes before rinsing.
- **Benefits**: Relieves bloating and soothes muscle spasms.
- **Personal Note**: After a heavy meal, this remedy feels like a lifesaver.

2. IBS Relief Formula

- **What You'll Need:**
    - 50% DMSO solution
    - 1 teaspoon aloe vera gel
    - 2 drops chamomile essential oil
- **How to Use:**
    - Combine the ingredients in a glass container.
    - Apply a thin layer to the abdomen and massage gently.
    - Allow it to absorb fully; no rinsing needed.
- **Benefits**: Reduces inflammation and calms digestive discomfort.

3. SIBO Support Spray

- **What You'll Need:**
    - 50% DMSO solution
    - 1 teaspoon distilled water
    - 3 drops oregano essential oil
- **How to Use:**
    - Combine ingredients in a glass spray bottle.
    - Shake well and spray onto the abdomen.
    - Massage in gently for even application.
- **Benefits**: Combats harmful bacteria while soothing the gut.

4. Constipation Relief Massage

- **What You'll Need:**
    - 50% DMSO solution
    - 1 teaspoon castor oil

- **How to Use:**
  - Mix the ingredients thoroughly.
  - Massage onto the lower abdomen in gentle, clockwise motions.
  - Allow it to absorb for 30 minutes before rinsing.
- **Benefits**: Promotes bowel movement and eases discomfort.
- **Personal Note**: This has become a trusted part of my routine during those stubborn weeks.

5. Aloe and DMSO Gut Soother

- **What You'll Need:**
  - 50% DMSO solution
  - 1 tablespoon aloe vera gel
- **How to Use:**
  - Mix the DMSO and aloe vera gel.
  - Apply to the abdomen and let it absorb.
  - Reapply daily for consistent relief.
- **Benefits**: Hydrates and repairs the gut lining.

6. Ginger and DMSO Digestive Tea

- **What You'll Need:**
  - 1/4 teaspoon food-grade DMSO (diluted to 10%)
  - 1 cup hot water
  - 1 teaspoon grated ginger
- **How to Use:**
  - Steep the ginger in hot water for 5 minutes.
  - Add the DMSO once the tea has cooled slightly.
  - Sip slowly to soothe the gut and promote digestion.

- **Benefits**: Combines ginger's digestive support with DMSO's cellular repair.

7. Detoxifying Gut Soak

    - **What You'll Need:**
        - 1/4 cup 50% DMSO solution
        - Warm water (enough to fill a basin)
    - **How to Use:**
        - Add DMSO to a basin of warm water.
        - Soak your feet for 20 minutes while relaxing.
        - Rinse and pat dry.
    - **Benefits**: Promotes detoxification and supports gut health through systemic effects.

8. Leaky Gut Repair Blend

    - **What You'll Need:**
        - 50% DMSO solution
        - 1/4 teaspoon powdered glutamine
        - 1 teaspoon distilled water
    - **How to Use:**
        - Dissolve the glutamine in water and mix with DMSO.
        - Apply to the abdomen using clean hands or a cotton pad.
        - Let it absorb for 20–30 minutes before rinsing.
    - **Benefits**: Supports gut barrier repair and reduces inflammation.

Tips for Digestive Health

- **Stay Hydrated**: Water aids digestion and complements DMSO's effects.
- **Focus on Nutrition**: Pair DMSO remedies with a diet rich in fiber, probiotics, and anti-inflammatory foods.
- **Listen to Your Body**: Track your symptoms and adjust remedies as needed.

Finding Balance with DMSO

Digestive challenges can feel isolating, but you're not alone—and you have options. These DMSO remedies provide practical, effective ways to manage symptoms, repair damage, and restore balance to your gut. With time and consistency, you'll find that comfort and confidence are well within reach.

In the next section, we'll explore how DMSO can support detoxification, expanding its role in holistic healing.

8.2 Internal Detox: Heavy Metals and Cellular Detoxification

Our bodies face daily exposure to toxins—from heavy metals in the environment to chemicals in processed foods and household products. Over time, these toxins can accumulate, straining the body's natural detox systems and affecting overall health. I've felt the weight of this myself—fatigue, brain fog, and a sense that something wasn't quite right. That's when I turned to DMSO for detoxification, and the results were nothing short of transformative.

DMSO's ability to bind with and remove toxins makes it an invaluable tool for supporting the body's natural detox processes. Let's explore how this multitasking molecule can help you eliminate harmful substances and restore balance.

Why DMSO Works for Detoxification

DMSO's detoxifying properties come from its unique chemistry:

- **Heavy Metal Binding**: Forms complexes with toxic metals like mercury, lead, and aluminum, aiding their removal from the body.
- **Cellular Transport**: Delivers antioxidants and nutrients to cells while flushing out toxins.
- **Antioxidant Action**: Neutralizes free radicals, reducing oxidative stress and protecting cells.

10+ Remedies for Internal Detox

1. General Detox Drink

- **What You'll Need:**
    - 1/4 teaspoon food-grade DMSO (diluted to 10%)
    - 1 cup distilled water
    - Juice of 1/2 lemon
- **How to Use:**
    - Combine all ingredients in a glass container.
    - Drink slowly, preferably on an empty stomach.
    - Follow with a glass of plain water.
- **Benefits**: Supports systemic detox and boosts overall cellular health.

2. Heavy Metal Chelation Blend

- **What You'll Need:**
    - 1/4 teaspoon food-grade DMSO (diluted to 10%)
    - 1 cup distilled water
    - 1/4 teaspoon cilantro juice
- **How to Use:**
    - Mix the ingredients in a glass container.
    - Sip slowly, once daily, for up to two weeks.
    - Follow with a high-fiber diet to support elimination.
- **Benefits**: Combines DMSO's binding properties with cilantro's heavy metal detox effects.

3. Liver Cleanse Protocol

- **What You'll Need:**
    - 1/4 teaspoon food-grade DMSO (diluted to 10%)
    - 1 teaspoon milk thistle extract
    - 1 cup warm water
- **How to Use:**
    - Mix all ingredients thoroughly.
    - Drink once daily, preferably in the morning.
    - Continue for two weeks, then take a break for one week.
- **Benefits**: Enhances liver function and promotes the removal of toxins.

4. Antioxidant Detox Tea

- **What You'll Need:**
    - 1/4 teaspoon food-grade DMSO (diluted to 10%)
    - 1 cup green tea (brewed and cooled)

- **How to Use:**
  - Add DMSO to the cooled green tea.
  - Sip slowly to allow absorption.
  - Use 2–3 times a week for ongoing support.
- **Benefits**: Combines green tea's antioxidant properties with DMSO's cellular detox effects.

5. Colon Cleanse Formula

- **What You'll Need:**
  - 1/4 teaspoon food-grade DMSO (diluted to 10%)
  - 1 teaspoon psyllium husk
  - 1 cup distilled water
- **How to Use:**
  - Mix the ingredients and drink immediately.
  - Follow with an additional glass of water.
  - Use once daily for up to one week.
- **Benefits**: Supports bowel regularity and removes toxins from the digestive tract.

6. Kidney Support Tonic

- **What You'll Need:**
  - 1/4 teaspoon food-grade DMSO (diluted to 10%)
  - 1 cup cranberry juice (unsweetened)
- **How to Use:**
  - Mix the DMSO with the cranberry juice.
  - Drink once daily for up to one week.

- **Benefits**: Flushes toxins from the kidneys while supporting urinary tract health.

7. **Skin Detoxification Spray**

    - **What You'll Need:**
        - 50% DMSO solution
        - 1 tablespoon distilled water
        - 3 drops tea tree oil

    - **How to Use:**
        - Combine ingredients in a glass spray bottle.
        - Spray onto areas prone to toxin buildup, like the feet or underarms.
        - Let it air dry; no rinsing needed.

    - **Benefits**: Promotes toxin release through the skin.

8. **Lymphatic Detox Wrap**

    - **What You'll Need:**
        - 50% DMSO solution
        - Soft cloth or gauze
        - Elastic bandage

    - **How to Use:**
        - Soak the cloth in DMSO and wrap it around the lymphatic areas (e.g., armpits, neck).
        - Secure with an elastic bandage and leave on for 1–2 hours.
        - Remove and rinse the area with cool water.

    - **Benefits**: Supports lymphatic drainage and detoxification.

Tips for Detox Success

- **Stay Hydrated**: Drink plenty of water to help flush toxins through the kidneys and bladder.
- **Start Slow**: Begin with lower doses to allow your body to adjust.
- **Pair with Nutritional Support**: Incorporate a diet rich in antioxidants, fiber, and detoxifying foods like leafy greens and cruciferous vegetables.

A Clean Slate with DMSO

Detoxification isn't just about eliminating toxins—it's about creating a foundation for better health. With these DMSO remedies, you can support your body's natural processes, restore balance, and feel revitalized from the inside out. Whether you're tackling heavy metals or simply seeking a gentle reset, these solutions provide practical, accessible steps toward a cleaner, healthier you.

In the next section, we'll explore how DMSO pairs with natural detox agents for even greater benefits.

8.3 Pairing DMSO with Natural Detox Agents

Detoxification is a powerful way to support your body's health, and when you combine DMSO with natural detox agents, the results can be transformative. From heavy metals to environmental toxins, this combination helps your body eliminate harmful substances more efficiently while delivering nutrients and antioxidants directly to the cells that need them most. When I first tried pairing DMSO with natural agents like activated charcoal and green tea, I was amazed at how much more energized and clear-headed I felt. These combinations are simple yet effective, making them an essential part of any detox routine.

Why Combine DMSO with Natural Detox Agents?

DMSO is a carrier molecule, meaning it enhances the absorption and effectiveness of other substances. By pairing it with detox agents, you amplify their benefits while targeting toxins at a deeper level. Here's why it works:

- **Enhanced Absorption**: Delivers detox agents directly into cells and tissues.
- **Synergistic Effects**: Combines the unique properties of DMSO with the benefits of natural detox agents like antioxidants and chelators.
- **Comprehensive Detox**: Targets multiple pathways, from binding toxins in the gut to supporting liver and kidney function.

10+ Remedies for Enhanced Detoxification

1. Activated Charcoal and DMSO Blend

- **What You'll Need:**
    - 50% DMSO solution
    - 1/4 teaspoon activated charcoal powder
    - 1 teaspoon distilled water
- **How to Use:**
    - Mix the charcoal powder with distilled water to form a paste.
    - Add the DMSO and mix thoroughly.
    - Apply to the abdomen or lower back and let it absorb for 20–30 minutes.
    - Rinse with cool water.
- **Benefits**: Binds toxins in the digestive tract while supporting systemic detox.

2. Cilantro and DMSO Detox Wrap

- **What You'll Need:**
  - 50% DMSO solution
  - 1 teaspoon fresh cilantro juice
  - Soft gauze or cloth
- **How to Use:**
  - Combine the DMSO and cilantro juice.
  - Soak the gauze in the mixture and wrap around the wrists or ankles.
  - Leave on for 30 minutes before removing.
- **Benefits**: Combines cilantro's heavy metal chelation properties with DMSO's transport abilities.

3. Green Tea and DMSO Antioxidant Mist

- **What You'll Need:**
  - 50% DMSO solution
  - 1 tablespoon brewed green tea (cooled)
  - Glass spray bottle
- **How to Use:**
  - Mix the ingredients in the spray bottle.
  - Spray onto the skin, focusing on areas with good circulation (e.g., wrists, neck).
  - Let it air dry; no rinsing needed.
- **Benefits**: Combines the antioxidant power of green tea with DMSO's deep tissue action.

4. Milk Thistle and DMSO Liver Support

- **What You'll Need:**
    - 50% DMSO solution
    - 1 teaspoon milk thistle extract
    - 1 cup warm water
- **How to Use:**
    - Mix the milk thistle extract and warm water.
    - Add the DMSO and stir gently.
    - Apply to the abdomen over the liver and let it absorb for 20–30 minutes.
- **Benefits**: Supports liver detoxification and promotes cell repair.

5. Epsom Salt and DMSO Skin Soak

- **What You'll Need:**
    - 1/4 cup 50% DMSO solution
    - 1 cup Epsom salts
    - Warm water (enough to fill a basin)
- **How to Use:**
    - Dissolve the Epsom salts in the warm water.
    - Add the DMSO and mix well.
    - Soak your feet or hands for 20 minutes.
- **Benefits**: Draws out toxins through the skin while replenishing magnesium levels.

6. Cranberry and DMSO Kidney Flush

- **What You'll Need:**
    o 1/4 teaspoon food-grade DMSO (diluted to 10%)
    o 1 cup unsweetened cranberry juice
- **How to Use:**
    o Mix the DMSO with cranberry juice.
    o Drink slowly, preferably in the morning.
    o Repeat for 3–5 days.
- **Benefits**: Flushes toxins from the kidneys and supports urinary health.

7. Bentonite Clay and DMSO Mask

- **What You'll Need:**
    o 50% DMSO solution
    o 1 teaspoon bentonite clay
    o 1 teaspoon distilled water
- **How to Use:**
    o Mix the bentonite clay with water to form a paste.
    o Add the DMSO and mix thoroughly.
    o Apply to the face or other targeted areas and leave for 15–20 minutes.
    o Rinse with warm water.
- **Benefits**: Draws out impurities and detoxifies the skin.

8. Vitamin C and DMSO Cellular Cleanse

- **What You'll Need:**
  - 50% DMSO solution
  - 1/4 teaspoon powdered vitamin C
  - 1 teaspoon distilled water

- **How to Use:**
  - Dissolve the vitamin C in water.
  - Mix with DMSO and apply to the wrists or inner forearms.
  - Let it absorb for 20 minutes before rinsing.

- **Benefits**: Neutralizes free radicals and promotes collagen repair.

Tips for Combining DMSO with Detox Agents

- **Start Slow**: Begin with lower concentrations of DMSO and natural agents to avoid overwhelming your system.
- **Hydrate Well**: Drink plenty of water to support toxin elimination through the kidneys and bladder.
- **Track Your Progress**: Keep a journal of symptoms and results to refine your detox regimen.

A Powerful Detox Partnership

DMSO and natural detox agents form a powerful team, working together to eliminate toxins, restore balance, and enhance your overall health. These remedies offer a practical and effective way to harness the best of both worlds, making detoxification a more accessible and transformative process.

In the next chapter, we'll explore how DMSO can support joint and bone health, addressing conditions like arthritis and osteoporosis.

Chapter 9

BONE AND JOINT HEALTH

9.1 Remedies for Osteoarthritis and Joint Mobility

Joint health plays a vital role in maintaining mobility and independence, but conditions like osteoarthritis can make even the simplest tasks feel insurmountable. I've seen loved ones grapple with the stiffness and discomfort of arthritis—the slow, frustrating limitation it places on daily life. Watching their struggle motivated me to explore solutions that didn't just mask the symptoms but addressed the root causes. That's where DMSO became a game-changer.

DMSO's unique ability to reduce inflammation, enhance blood flow, and support tissue repair makes it a natural choice for managing osteoarthritis and improving joint mobility. These remedies, combined with consistency and care, offer a way to ease discomfort and regain freedom of movement.

Why DMSO is Effective for Osteoarthritis

Osteoarthritis is caused by the breakdown of cartilage, leading to inflammation, pain, and stiffness in the joints. DMSO tackles these issues through:

- **Anti-Inflammatory Action**: Reduces swelling and discomfort in affected joints.
- **Pain Relief**: Blocks pain signals for near-instant relief.
- **Tissue Support**: Promotes cellular repair and improves joint lubrication.

10+ Remedies for Osteoarthritis and Joint Mobility

1. Topical Pain Relief Rub

- **What You'll Need:**
    - 70% DMSO solution
    - 1 teaspoon magnesium oil
    - 2 drops peppermint essential oil
- **How to Use:**
    - Mix ingredients in a small glass container.
    - Massage gently into the affected joint using clean hands.
    - Let it absorb for 20–30 minutes before rinsing.
- **Benefits**: Reduces inflammation and soothes aching joints.
- **Personal Note**: This blend is my dad's favorite for his hands after gardening—simple yet effective.

2. Warm Joint Mobility Compress

- **What You'll Need:**
    - 50% DMSO solution
    - Warm, damp towel

- **How to Use:**
    - Apply DMSO to the joint with a cotton pad.
    - Cover the area with the warm towel for 15–20 minutes.
    - Remove the towel and let the skin air dry.

- **Benefits**: Loosens stiff joints and enhances circulation.

3. Turmeric and DMSO Anti-Inflammatory Paste

- **What You'll Need:**
    - 50% DMSO solution
    - 1/2 teaspoon turmeric powder
    - 1 teaspoon distilled water

- **How to Use:**
    - Mix the turmeric with water to form a paste.
    - Add DMSO and stir thoroughly.
    - Apply to the joint and leave for 15 minutes before rinsing.

- **Benefits**: Combines turmeric's anti-inflammatory properties with DMSO's tissue-penetrating action.

4. Epsom Salt and DMSO Joint Soak

- **What You'll Need:**
    - 1/4 cup 50% DMSO solution
    - 1 cup Epsom salts
    - Warm water (enough to fill a basin)

- **How to Use:**
  - Dissolve Epsom salts in the warm water.
  - Add DMSO and mix well.
  - Soak the affected joint for 20 minutes.
  - Pat dry after soaking.
- **Benefits**: Reduces swelling and relaxes tight tissues.

5. Overnight Joint Relief Wrap

- **What You'll Need:**
  - 70% DMSO solution
  - Soft gauze or cloth
  - Elastic bandage
- **How to Use:**
  - Soak the gauze in DMSO and wrap it around the joint.
  - Secure with an elastic bandage and leave on overnight.
  - Remove in the morning and rinse the area.
- **Benefits**: Provides sustained relief and promotes healing during sleep.

6. Collagen-Boosting Massage Oil

- **What You'll Need:**
  - 50% DMSO solution
  - 1 teaspoon collagen powder
  - 1 teaspoon olive oil
- **How to Use:**
  - Mix the ingredients thoroughly.
  - Massage gently into the joint and let it absorb for 30 minutes.
  - Rinse if necessary.

- **Benefits**: Supports joint lubrication and cartilage repair.

7. Cooling Relief Gel

- **What You'll Need:**
    - 50% DMSO solution
    - 1 tablespoon aloe vera gel
    - 2 drops peppermint essential oil
- **How to Use:**
    - Combine ingredients in a glass container.
    - Apply a thin layer to the joint and let it absorb fully.
    - Reapply as needed for ongoing relief.
- **Personal Note**: This gel feels amazing after a long walk or hike—refreshing and soothing.

8. Anti-Stiffness Lotion

- **What You'll Need:**
    - 50% DMSO solution
    - 1 teaspoon shea butter
    - 1 drop lavender essential oil
- **How to Use:**
    - Melt the shea butter slightly to soften it.
    - Mix with DMSO and lavender oil.
    - Massage into stiff joints twice daily.
- **Benefits**: Hydrates the skin while easing stiffness and pain.

Tips for Improving Joint Mobility

- **Stay Active**: Gentle exercises like yoga or swimming complement DMSO remedies and keep joints flexible.
- **Consistency Matters**: Regular application is key to managing chronic conditions like osteoarthritis.
- **Listen to Your Body**: Adjust remedies based on your comfort level and specific needs.

Regaining Mobility, One Step at a Time

Osteoarthritis doesn't have to limit your life. With DMSO, you have a practical, powerful tool to manage pain, reduce inflammation, and restore flexibility. These remedies are designed to support your joints, helping you move through life with greater ease and confidence.

In the next section, we'll explore how DMSO can support bone health, including its role in fracture recovery and strengthening.

9.2 Bone Strengthening and Recovery from Fractures

Bones are remarkable—they carry us through life's adventures, withstand wear and tear, and heal themselves when fractured. But the process of bone healing can be slow and painful, especially for injuries like fractures, stress fractures, or even bone-related conditions like osteoporosis. When my cousin broke her ankle, she was frustrated with the long recovery time and the discomfort that came with it. That's when I introduced her to DMSO, and she was amazed at how it complemented her recovery.

DMSO enhances bone healing by reducing inflammation, improving circulation, and delivering nutrients directly to the site of injury. Whether you're recovering from a fracture or looking to strengthen your bones, these remedies can help support and accelerate the healing process.

Why DMSO Works for Bone Health

Bone healing requires a delicate balance of inflammation, cellular repair, and nutrient delivery. DMSO supports this process in several ways:

- **Anti-Inflammatory**: Reduces swelling and pain at the injury site.
- **Circulation Booster**: Enhances blood flow, delivering oxygen and nutrients to support bone repair.
- **Carrier Molecule**: Transports calcium, magnesium, and other essential nutrients directly to the bones.

10+ Remedies for Bone Healing

1. Topical Fracture Relief Rub

- **What You'll Need:**
    - 70% DMSO solution
    - 1 teaspoon magnesium oil
- **How to Use:**
    - Mix the DMSO with magnesium oil.
    - Massage gently around the fracture site (not on open wounds).
    - Allow it to absorb for 20–30 minutes before rinsing.
- **Benefits**: Reduces inflammation and supports muscle relaxation around the injury.

2. DMSO and Calcium Topical Blend

- **What You'll Need:**
    - 50% DMSO solution
    - 1/4 teaspoon calcium powder
    - 1 teaspoon distilled water
- **How to Use:**
    - Dissolve the calcium powder in water.
    - Mix with DMSO and apply to the injured area.
    - Let it absorb fully, then rinse.
- **Benefits**: Enhances calcium delivery to support bone strength and repair.

3. Anti-Inflammatory Bone Healing Compress

- **What You'll Need:**
    - 70% DMSO solution
    - Warm, damp towel
- **How to Use:**
    - Apply DMSO to the affected area using a cotton pad.
    - Cover with the warm towel and leave for 15–20 minutes.
    - Remove and let the area air dry.
- **Benefits**: Reduces swelling and promotes blood flow to the injury.

4. Bone Healing Foot Soak

- **What You'll Need:**
    - 1/4 cup 50% DMSO solution
    - 1 cup Epsom salts
    - Warm water (enough to fill a basin)

- **How to Use:**
  - Dissolve Epsom salts in the warm water.
  - Add DMSO and mix well.
  - Soak the affected foot or ankle for 20 minutes.
- **Benefits**: Relieves pain and inflammation while promoting healing.

5. Collagen-Boosting Topical Serum

- **What You'll Need:**
  - 50% DMSO solution
  - 1/4 teaspoon collagen powder
  - 1 teaspoon olive oil
- **How to Use:**
  - Mix the collagen powder with olive oil, then add DMSO.
  - Massage gently around the injury site.
  - Let it absorb for 20--30 minutes before rinsing.
- **Benefits**: Supports connective tissue and bone strength.

6. Overnight Bone Healing Wrap

- **What You'll Need:**
  - 70% DMSO solution
  - Soft cloth or gauze
  - Elastic bandage
- **How to Use:**
  - Soak the cloth in DMSO and wrap around the injured area.
  - Secure with an elastic bandage and leave overnight.
  - Remove in the morning and rinse the area.
- **Benefits**: Provides sustained support for long-term healing.

7. DMSO and Turmeric Bone Healing Paste

- **What You'll Need:**
  - 50% DMSO solution
  - 1/2 teaspoon turmeric powder
  - 1 teaspoon distilled water
- **How to Use:**
  - Mix turmeric with water to form a paste, then add DMSO.
  - Apply to the area and leave for 15–20 minutes before rinsing.
- **Benefits**: Combines turmeric's anti-inflammatory properties with DMSO's tissue-penetrating action.

8. Nutrient-Enhanced Bone Drink

- **What You'll Need:**
  - 1/4 teaspoon food-grade DMSO (diluted to 10%)
  - 1 cup almond milk
  - 1/4 teaspoon powdered calcium and magnesium blend
- **How to Use:**
  - Mix the ingredients thoroughly.
  - Drink once daily for two weeks, then take a one-week break.
- **Benefits**: Supports bone mineralization and systemic healing.

Tips for Supporting Bone Healing

- **Be Patient**: Bone healing takes time—use DMSO consistently for best results.
- **Support with Nutrition**: Include bone-healthy foods like leafy greens, nuts, and seeds in your diet.

- **Gentle Movement**: Engage in low-impact exercises to promote circulation and prevent stiffness.

Building Stronger Bones with DMSO

Bone injuries may take time to heal, but with DMSO, you have a tool to accelerate the process and reduce discomfort along the way. These remedies are designed to complement your body's natural ability to repair itself, giving you the support you need to regain strength and mobility.

In the next section, we'll explore how DMSO can be combined with joint supplements to further enhance its benefits.

9.3 Managing Chronic Inflammation in Joints

When it comes to joint health, DMSO is a powerful ally on its own. But when paired with targeted joint supplements like glucosamine, chondroitin, and collagen, its benefits are amplified. These combinations not only relieve pain and inflammation but also address the root causes of joint issues, such as cartilage breakdown and loss of flexibility. I've seen the transformative effects of these blends firsthand—whether it was helping a friend bounce back from a knee injury or improving my own post-workout stiffness.

By combining DMSO with supplements, you're not just soothing discomfort—you're giving your joints the building blocks they need to heal and thrive.

Why DMSO Enhances Joint Supplements

DMSO's role as a carrier molecule allows it to transport supplements directly to the affected area, increasing their bioavailability and effectiveness. Here's why this synergy works:

- **Enhanced Delivery**: Ensures supplements like glucosamine and MSM reach deep into joint tissues.
- **Anti-Inflammatory**: Combats swelling and pain, complementing the healing properties of supplements.
- **Support for Cartilage Repair**: Works alongside joint supplements to rebuild and maintain cartilage.

10+ Remedies for Combining DMSO with Joint Supplements

1. Glucosamine and DMSO Topical Blend

- **What You'll Need:**
    - 50% DMSO solution
    - 1/4 teaspoon powdered glucosamine sulfate
    - 1 teaspoon distilled water
- **How to Use:**
    - Dissolve the glucosamine sulfate in water.
    - Mix with DMSO and apply to the affected joint.
    - Let it absorb for 20–30 minutes before rinsing.
- **Benefits**: Supports cartilage repair and reduces inflammation.

2. Chondroitin and DMSO Joint Rub

- **What You'll Need:**
    - 50% DMSO solution
    - 1/4 teaspoon powdered chondroitin sulfate
    - 1 teaspoon olive oil
- **How to Use:**
    - Mix the chondroitin with olive oil, then add DMSO.

- o Massage into the joint, focusing on sore areas.
- o Allow it to absorb fully; no rinsing needed.
- **Benefits**: Improves joint lubrication and mobility.

3. Collagen and DMSO Healing Serum

- **What You'll Need:**
  - o 50% DMSO solution
  - o 1/4 teaspoon powdered collagen
  - o 1 teaspoon aloe vera gel
- **How to Use:**
  - o Mix the collagen with aloe vera gel, then add DMSO.
  - o Apply a thin layer to the joint and let it absorb for 20–30 minutes.
  - o Reapply daily for best results.
- **Benefits**: Supports connective tissue repair and strengthens cartilage.

4. MSM and DMSO Anti-Inflammatory Paste

- **What You'll Need:**
  - o 50% DMSO solution
  - o 1/4 teaspoon powdered MSM (methylsulfonylmethane)
  - o 1 teaspoon distilled water
- **How to Use:**
  - o Dissolve MSM in water, then mix with DMSO.
  - o Apply to the joint and let it absorb for 20 minutes.
  - o Rinse if necessary.
- **Benefits**: Reduces inflammation and enhances joint flexibility.

5. Turmeric and DMSO Joint Gel

- **What You'll Need:**
    - 50% DMSO solution
    - 1/2 teaspoon turmeric powder
    - 1 teaspoon coconut oil
- **How to Use:**
    - Mix turmeric and coconut oil into a paste, then add DMSO.
    - Apply to the joint and let it sit for 15–20 minutes.
    - Rinse with warm water.
- **Benefits**: Combines anti-inflammatory properties with joint repair.

6. Multisupplement Joint Health Wrap

- **What You'll Need:**
    - 70% DMSO solution
    - 1/4 teaspoon glucosamine, chondroitin, and MSM powder blend
    - Soft gauze or cloth
    - Elastic bandage
- **How to Use:**
    - Mix the powder blend with DMSO.
    - Soak the gauze in the mixture and wrap around the joint.
    - Secure with the elastic bandage and leave on for 1–2 hours.
    - Remove and rinse the area.
- **Benefits**: Provides sustained delivery of multiple joint-supporting nutrients.

7. Epsom Salt and DMSO Foot Soak

- **What You'll Need:**
    - 1/4 cup 50% DMSO solution
    - 1 cup Epsom salts
    - Warm water (enough to fill a basin)
- **How to Use:**
    - Dissolve Epsom salts in warm water, then add DMSO.
    - Soak the affected joint for 20 minutes.
    - Pat dry after soaking.
- **Benefits**: Relieves pain and swelling while delivering magnesium to support joint health.

8. Recovery Drink for Joint Health

- **What You'll Need:**
    - 1/4 teaspoon food-grade DMSO (diluted to 10%)
    - 1 cup almond milk
    - 1/4 teaspoon collagen powder
    - 1/4 teaspoon powdered glucosamine sulfate
- **How to Use:**
    - Mix all ingredients thoroughly.
    - Drink once daily for two weeks, then take a one-week break.
- **Benefits**: Supports joint health from the inside out.

Tips for Combining DMSO with Supplements

- **Start Slow**: Begin with lower concentrations to allow your body to adjust.

- **Be Consistent**: Regular application and use of supplements yield the best results.
- **Listen to Your Body**: Adjust remedies based on your comfort and specific needs.

Strengthening Joints, Enhancing Mobility

Combining DMSO with joint supplements creates a powerful synergy that supports joint health from every angle. These remedies don't just relieve pain—they help rebuild and maintain your joints, giving you the freedom to move with confidence and ease.

In the next chapter, we'll explore how DMSO can be combined with natural remedies to enhance its versatility and benefits.

Part IV

ADVANCED APPLICATIONS

Chapter 10

COMBINING DMSO WITH OTHER THERAPIES

10.1 Essential Oils for Enhanced Relief

Essential oils have been treasured for centuries for their healing properties, from calming lavender to invigorating peppermint. When paired with DMSO, these oils become even more potent, delivering their benefits deeply and effectively. DMSO enhances absorption, ensuring essential oils target the precise areas where they're needed most. From relieving pain to promoting relaxation, this synergy opens up endless possibilities for natural healing.

Why Combine DMSO with Essential Oils?

The combination of DMSO and essential oils creates powerful remedies by:

- **Deep Penetration**: DMSO drives essential oils directly into tissues for faster, targeted relief.
- **Synergistic Effects**: Enhances the therapeutic properties of essential oils by amplifying their effectiveness.
- **Customizable Solutions**: Easily tailored blends for specific conditions, such as pain, inflammation, or stress.

10+ Unique Remedies with DMSO and Essential Oils

1. Lavender and DMSO for Restful Sleep

- What You'll Need:
  - 50% DMSO solution
  - 3 drops lavender essential oil
  - 1 teaspoon aloe vera gel
- How to Use:
  - Mix the ingredients in a glass container.
  - Apply to the back of your neck and wrists before bedtime.
  - Massage gently and let it absorb fully.
- **Benefits**: Promotes relaxation and supports deeper sleep.

2. Helichrysum and DMSO for Scar Healing

- What You'll Need:
  - 50% DMSO solution
  - 3 drops helichrysum essential oil
  - 1 teaspoon vitamin E oil

- **How to Use:**
  - Combine ingredients in a small container.
  - Massage onto scars or healing wounds (only on closed wounds).
  - Use daily for improved skin texture and reduced scarring.
- **Benefits**: Accelerates scar healing and reduces discoloration.

3. Peppermint and DMSO for Digestive Relief

- **What You'll Need:**
  - 50% DMSO solution
  - 2 drops peppermint essential oil
  - 1 teaspoon magnesium oil
- **How to Use:**
  - Mix the ingredients thoroughly.
  - Apply to the abdomen using a cotton pad.
  - Massage gently and let it absorb for 20–30 minutes.
- **Benefits**: Eases bloating and soothes abdominal discomfort.

4. Eucalyptus and DMSO for Sinus Congestion

- **What You'll Need:**
  - 50% DMSO solution
  - 3 drops eucalyptus essential oil
  - 1 teaspoon distilled water
- **How to Use:**
  - Mix ingredients in a glass spray bottle.
  - Spray lightly over your chest and upper back.
  - Massage gently for even coverage.
- **Benefits**: Opens airways and clears nasal passages.

5. Tea Tree and DMSO for Acne Relief

- **What You'll Need:**
  - 50% DMSO solution
  - 2 drops tea tree essential oil
  - Cotton swab

- **How to Use:**
  - Combine DMSO and tea tree oil in a small container.
  - Dip a cotton swab into the mixture and apply directly to blemishes.
  - Let it absorb for 10–15 minutes before rinsing.

- **Benefits**: Reduces inflammation and prevents acne-causing bacteria.

6. Rosemary and DMSO for Hair Growth

- **What You'll Need:**
  - 50% DMSO solution
  - 3 drops rosemary essential oil
  - 1 tablespoon aloe vera gel

- **How to Use:**
  - Mix the ingredients into a smooth gel.
  - Massage into your scalp and leave for 30 minutes.
  - Rinse thoroughly with warm water.

- **Benefits**: Stimulates hair growth and improves scalp health.

7. Clary Sage and DMSO for Hormonal Balance

- **What You'll Need:**
  - 50% DMSO solution
  - 2 drops clary sage essential oil
  - 1 teaspoon coconut oil

- **How to Use:**
  - Combine ingredients in a glass container.
  - Apply to the lower abdomen and massage gently.
  - Let it absorb fully; no rinsing needed.
- **Benefits**: Eases hormonal discomfort and supports balance.

8. Bergamot and DMSO for Stress Relief

- **What You'll Need:**
  - 50% DMSO solution
  - 3 drops bergamot essential oil
  - 1 teaspoon olive oil
- **How to Use:**
  - Mix the ingredients thoroughly.
  - Apply to your wrists or temples for calming effects.
  - Let it absorb fully; no rinsing needed.
- **Benefits**: Reduces stress and promotes a positive mood.

9. Lemongrass and DMSO for Muscle Pain

- **What You'll Need:**
  - 50% DMSO solution
  - 2 drops lemongrass essential oil
  - 1 teaspoon magnesium oil
- **How to Use:**
  - Mix ingredients thoroughly and apply to sore muscles.
  - Massage in circular motions and let it absorb.
  - Rinse if necessary.
- **Benefits**: Relieves soreness and reduces muscle tension.

Tips for Combining DMSO with Essential Oils

- **Start Small**: Essential oils are potent; always use a small amount when mixing with DMSO.
- **Patch Test First**: Test a small area to check for sensitivity before applying widely.
- **Dilute Properly**: Use appropriate dilution ratios for essential oils to prevent irritation.

A Dynamic Healing Duo

The combination of DMSO and essential oils creates versatile, highly effective remedies for a variety of health needs. These blends are not only practical but also easy to tailor, ensuring you have the perfect solution for everything from pain relief to emotional well-being. With these recipes, you can unlock the full potential of natural healing.

In the next section, we'll explore how DMSO pairs with herbal remedies to further enhance its versatility.

10.2 Pairing DMSO with Herbal Remedies

Herbs have been a cornerstone of natural healing for centuries, offering diverse benefits for the body and mind. When combined with DMSO, these herbal remedies become even more effective, targeting issues like inflammation, stress, and skin repair with enhanced precision. The result is a dynamic synergy that leverages the best of nature and science.

Let's explore unique, innovative herbal and DMSO combinations that go beyond the remedies we've previously discussed.

Why Combine DMSO with Herbal Remedies?

DMSO complements herbal remedies by enhancing absorption, targeting delivery, and amplifying their therapeutic effects. This makes herbal extracts, tinctures, and powders more effective in addressing specific health concerns.

10+ Unique Remedies with DMSO and Herbal Remedies

1. Licorice Root and DMSO for Digestive Relief

- What You'll Need:
    - 50% DMSO solution
    - 1 teaspoon licorice root tea (cooled)
- How to Use:
    - Brew licorice root tea and let it cool.
    - Mix with DMSO and apply to the abdomen using a cotton pad.
    - Let it absorb fully; no rinsing needed.
- **Benefits**: Soothes digestive discomfort and supports gut health.

2. Comfrey and DMSO for Bone Healing

- What You'll Need:
    - 50% DMSO solution
    - 1 teaspoon comfrey tincture
- How to Use:
    - Combine the DMSO and comfrey tincture.
    - Apply to areas of bone fractures or bruises using a clean applicator.
    - Let it absorb for 20–30 minutes before rinsing.
- **Benefits**: Supports bone repair and reduces swelling.

3. Dandelion and DMSO for Liver Support

- **What You'll Need:**
  - 50% DMSO solution
  - 1 teaspoon dandelion root extract
- **How to Use:**
  - Mix the DMSO with dandelion root extract in a small container.
  - Apply to the lower right abdomen (over the liver) using a cotton pad.
  - Let it absorb fully; no rinsing needed.
- **Benefits**: Enhances liver detoxification and supports cellular repair.

4. Marshmallow Root and DMSO for Skin Soothing

- **What You'll Need:**
  - 50% DMSO solution
  - 1 teaspoon marshmallow root tea (cooled)
- **How to Use:**
  - Brew marshmallow root tea and let it cool.
  - Mix with DMSO and apply to irritated or dry skin.
  - Reapply as needed throughout the day.
- **Benefits**: Hydrates and soothes dry, flaky, or irritated skin.

5. Ginkgo Biloba and DMSO for Circulation

- **What You'll Need:**
  - 50% DMSO solution
  - 1 teaspoon ginkgo biloba tincture

- **How to Use:**
  - Combine the DMSO with ginkgo biloba tincture.
  - Apply to areas with poor circulation, such as hands or feet.
  - Massage gently and let it absorb fully.
- **Benefits**: Stimulates blood flow and improves circulation.

6. Valerian and DMSO for Sleep Support

- **What You'll Need:**
  - 50% DMSO solution
  - 1 teaspoon valerian root tincture
- **How to Use:**
  - Mix the DMSO and valerian tincture in a glass container.
  - Apply to the wrists or back of the neck before bedtime.
  - Let it absorb fully; no rinsing needed.
- **Benefits**: Promotes relaxation and supports restful sleep.

7. Echinacea and DMSO for Immune Support

- **What You'll Need:**
  - 50% DMSO solution
  - 1 teaspoon echinacea tincture
- **How to Use:**
  - Combine the ingredients and apply to the wrists or chest.
  - Massage gently and let it absorb fully.
  - Use during cold and flu season for enhanced immunity.
- **Benefits**: Boosts immune function and reduces the severity of colds.

8. Horsetail and DMSO for Hair Health

- **What You'll Need:**
  - 50% DMSO solution
  - 1 teaspoon horsetail extract
  - 1 tablespoon aloe vera gel
- **How to Use:**
  - Mix the ingredients into a smooth gel.
  - Massage into the scalp and let it sit for 30 minutes.
  - Rinse thoroughly with warm water.
- **Benefits**: Strengthens hair follicles and supports scalp health.

9. Goldenrod and DMSO for Kidney Health

- **What You'll Need:**
  - 50% DMSO solution
  - 1 teaspoon goldenrod tincture
- **How to Use:**
  - Mix the DMSO with goldenrod tincture.
  - Apply to the lower back over the kidneys.
  - Let it absorb fully; no rinsing needed.
- **Benefits**: Supports kidney function and promotes detoxification.

Tips for Maximizing Results

- **Quality Herbs Matter**: Use high-quality tinctures, teas, or extracts for the best outcomes.
- **Storage**: Keep blends in amber glass bottles to preserve potency.
- **Start Small**: Always patch-test new combinations to ensure compatibility with your skin.

Nature's Power Enhanced by DMSO

Herbal remedies and DMSO form a potent team, offering targeted solutions for a wide range of health concerns. These unique combinations provide practical, natural ways to enhance your well-being, delivering the best of what nature and science have to offer.

In the next section, we'll explore how DMSO can amplify the effects of dietary supplements, unlocking even greater health benefits.

10.3 Supplements and DMSO for Targeted Benefits

Supplements play a critical role in modern health, offering targeted support for specific conditions, from inflammation to immune health. When paired with DMSO, these supplements become even more effective, delivered directly to the cells and tissues that need them most. Whether you're looking to reduce inflammation, boost energy, or improve skin and joint health, DMSO can elevate the power of your supplements to a new level.

Why Combine DMSO with Supplements?

DMSO enhances the benefits of supplements by:

- **Enhanced Absorption**: Transports nutrients directly into cells, bypassing digestive barriers.
- **Targeted Delivery**: Focuses supplements' effects on specific areas, such as joints, skin, or nerves.
- **Synergistic Effects**: Amplifies the therapeutic properties of vitamins, minerals, and other nutrients.

10+ Unique Remedies with DMSO and Supplements

1. Magnesium and DMSO for Muscle Relaxation

- **What You'll Need:**
    - 50% DMSO solution
    - 1 teaspoon magnesium oil
- **How to Use:**
    - Mix the ingredients in a small container.
    - Apply to sore muscles or cramping areas.
    - Massage gently and let it absorb for 20–30 minutes.
- **Benefits**: Relaxes muscles, reduces cramps, and improves circulation.

2. Vitamin C and DMSO for Immune Support

- **What You'll Need:**
    - 50% DMSO solution
    - 1/4 teaspoon powdered vitamin C
    - 1 teaspoon distilled water
- **How to Use:**
    - Dissolve the vitamin C in water, then mix with DMSO.
    - Apply to the wrists or inner forearms.
    - Let it absorb fully; no rinsing needed.
- **Benefits**: Enhances immune function and fights oxidative stress.

3. Zinc and DMSO for Skin Healing

- **What You'll Need:**
    - 50% DMSO solution
    - 1/4 teaspoon zinc sulfate powder
    - 1 teaspoon aloe vera gel

- **How to Use:**
  - Combine ingredients into a smooth gel.
  - Apply to wounds or irritated skin.
  - Reapply daily for improved healing.
- **Benefits**: Promotes skin repair and reduces inflammation.

4. Glutathione and DMSO for Detoxification

- **What You'll Need:**
  - 50% DMSO solution
  - 1/4 teaspoon powdered glutathione
  - 1 teaspoon distilled water
- **How to Use:**
  - Dissolve glutathione in water, then mix with DMSO.
  - Apply to the abdomen or lower back.
  - Let it absorb for 20–30 minutes.
- **Benefits**: Supports liver detoxification and cellular health.

5. CoQ10 and DMSO for Energy Support

- **What You'll Need:**
  - 50% DMSO solution
  - 1/4 teaspoon powdered CoQ10
  - 1 teaspoon olive oil
- **How to Use:**
  - Combine ingredients in a small container.
  - Apply to the chest or wrists using clean hands.
  - Let it absorb fully; no rinsing needed.
- **Benefits**: Boosts cellular energy and improves circulation.

6. Calcium and DMSO for Bone Health

- **What You'll Need:**
    - 50% DMSO solution
    - 1/4 teaspoon calcium powder
    - 1 teaspoon distilled water
- **How to Use:**
    - Dissolve calcium in water, then mix with DMSO.
    - Apply to areas with bone pain or fractures.
    - Let it absorb fully; no rinsing needed.
- **Benefits**: Supports bone repair and mineralization.

7. Collagen and DMSO for Joint and Skin Health

- **What You'll Need:**
    - 50% DMSO solution
    - 1/4 teaspoon powdered collagen
    - 1 teaspoon aloe vera gel
- **How to Use:**
    - Mix collagen with aloe vera gel, then add DMSO.
    - Apply to joints or skin for enhanced hydration and repair.
    - Reapply daily for best results.
- **Benefits**: Strengthens connective tissue and promotes youthful skin.

8. Turmeric and DMSO for Inflammation

- **What You'll Need:**
    - 50% DMSO solution
    - 1/4 teaspoon turmeric powder
    - 1 teaspoon distilled water

- **How to Use:**
  - Mix turmeric with water, then add DMSO.
  - Apply to areas of inflammation or stiffness.
  - Let it sit for 15–20 minutes before rinsing.
- **Benefits**: Combines turmeric's anti-inflammatory properties with DMSO's deep-tissue action.

9. MSM and DMSO for Joint Flexibility

- **What You'll Need:**
  - 50% DMSO solution
  - 1/4 teaspoon powdered MSM (methylsulfonylmethane)
  - 1 teaspoon distilled water
- **How to Use:**
  - Dissolve MSM in water, then mix with DMSO.
  - Apply to sore joints and let it absorb for 20 minutes.
  - Rinse if necessary.
- **Benefits**: Reduces joint pain and improves mobility.

10. Probiotics and DMSO for Gut Health

- **What You'll Need:**
  - 50% DMSO solution
  - 1/4 teaspoon powdered probiotics
  - 1 teaspoon distilled water
- **How to Use:**
  - Mix the probiotics with water, then add DMSO.
  - Apply to the abdomen for systemic absorption.
  - Use daily to support digestive health.

- **Benefits**: Enhances gut health and supports a balanced microbiome.

Tips for Combining DMSO with Supplements

- **Use Quality Supplements**: Choose high-quality powders or liquids for best results.
- **Start Slow**: Begin with smaller doses to monitor your body's response.
- **Target Problem Areas**: Apply remedies directly to affected areas for focused relief.

Unlocking Targeted Benefits with DMSO

The combination of DMSO and supplements creates a powerful synergy that enhances the absorption and efficacy of essential nutrients. Whether you're targeting inflammation, boosting immunity, or improving skin health, these remedies offer a practical and effective way to achieve your wellness goals.

In the next chapter, we'll explore how DMSO can be incorporated into daily routines for comprehensive health support.

CHAPTER 11

VETERINARY AND SPORTS MEDICINE

11.1 Applications for Animals: Safe Practices and Use Cases

When it comes to the healing power of DMSO, humans aren't the only beneficiaries. Animals, ranging from household pets to larger livestock, have also found relief through this versatile molecule. Whether you're addressing chronic joint pain in an aging dog, aiding a horse's recovery from a sprain, or supporting the overall well-being of your farm animals, DMSO can be a transformative tool. However, like any treatment, its use requires knowledge, care, and a clear understanding of proper practices.

Safe Practices for Using DMSO on Animals

1. Proper Dilution for Animal Use

Dilution is key to avoiding irritation or adverse effects. Animals typically have more sensitive skin than humans, so starting with a lower concentration—such as a 50% solution—ensures safety. For particularly sensitive areas, such as around wounds, even lower concentrations might be necessary.

2. Test Before Full Application

Animals cannot verbalize discomfort, so it's crucial to test a small area first. Apply a tiny amount of diluted DMSO to an inconspicuous spot and monitor for redness, swelling, or excessive discomfort over 24 hours.

3. Avoid Contaminants

DMSO's ability to penetrate the skin and carry substances into the body makes it critical to use only pharmaceutical-grade DMSO and ensure the application area is clean.

4. Frequency of Use

Animals metabolize substances differently than humans, so less frequent applications may suffice. Start with once daily and adjust as needed under the guidance of a veterinarian.

Use Cases for DMSO in Animals

1. Joint Pain and Arthritis Relief

Just as DMSO reduces inflammation and pain in humans, it can offer the same benefits for animals with arthritis or chronic joint issues. Gently massage a diluted solution into the affected joints, taking care to follow safe practices.

2. Soft Tissue Injuries

For sprains, strains, and muscle soreness, DMSO can reduce swelling and expedite healing. This makes it particularly popular in veterinary care for horses involved in equestrian sports.

3. Wound Care

DMSO's antimicrobial properties can help prevent infection and promote faster wound healing. Ensure wounds are cleaned thoroughly before application, as DMSO could otherwise carry contaminants into the tissue.

4. Skin Conditions

DMSO can alleviate localized itching, inflammation, or minor skin irritations in animals. However, avoid open sores or areas where skin integrity is compromised.

5. Respiratory Support for Livestock

Some studies and anecdotal reports suggest DMSO's potential in easing respiratory issues in livestock, particularly when combined with other veterinary treatments. Always consult a professional before considering this use.

A Word of Caution: Veterinary Oversight

While DMSO holds immense potential, veterinary oversight is essential for safe and effective use. Animals vary greatly in size, species, and sensitivity, and what works for one may not work for another. A veterinarian can guide dilution ratios, application methods, and appropriate use cases tailored to your animal's specific needs.

Personal Anecdote: Healing a Loyal Companion

When my aging Labrador began showing signs of arthritis, the joy of her once-bounding steps turned into a stiff, labored shuffle. After consulting her veterinarian, I incorporated a carefully diluted DMSO solution into her care routine, massaging it gently onto her aching joints. Within weeks, her mobility improved, and the light returned to her eyes as she once again chased squirrels in the backyard. Watching her rediscover her zest for life was a reminder of the profound impact DMSO can have—not just on humans but on the animals we hold dear.

11.2 Treating Injuries in High-Performance Athletes

Athletes push their bodies to the limit, and with intense performance comes an increased risk of injuries. DMSO has emerged as a go-to solution for high-performance athletes seeking effective relief from pain, inflammation, and recovery setbacks. Whether dealing with acute injuries or managing chronic conditions, DMSO can help athletes get back in the game with minimal downtime.

Why DMSO Appeals to Athletes

The properties that make DMSO effective for general injury treatment—its ability to reduce inflammation, alleviate pain, and expedite healing—are even more valuable for athletes who rely on quick recovery. For many, DMSO's versatility provides an edge in rehabilitation and performance optimization.

1. Rapid Absorption and Targeted Relief

DMSO penetrates the skin quickly, delivering pain relief and reducing swelling in localized areas. This is particularly useful for acute injuries like sprains or strains, where time is of the essence.

2. Safe for Repeated Use

Unlike some over-the-counter painkillers or corticosteroids, DMSO doesn't carry the same risks of dependency or systemic side effects when used topically. For athletes with recurring issues, this makes DMSO an attractive option.

Treating Common Sports Injuries with DMSO

1. Sprains and Strains

Athletes frequently suffer from overstretched ligaments or torn muscle fibers. Applying a diluted DMSO solution to the affected area can reduce swelling and pain, allowing for quicker return to training.

2. Tendonitis

Repetitive motions in sports like tennis, running, or weightlifting often lead to tendon inflammation. DMSO's anti-inflammatory properties can help soothe these flare-ups and improve mobility.

3. Bruising and Contusions

Impact injuries, whether from contact sports or accidental collisions, can result in painful bruising. DMSO accelerates the healing process by reducing inflammation and encouraging blood flow to the area.

4. Joint Pain from Overuse

Knees, shoulders, and elbows take a beating in high-performance sports. DMSO can offer relief for athletes managing chronic joint pain, enabling them to maintain their training schedules.

Enhancing Recovery with DMSO

DMSO isn't just for treating injuries—it's also a powerful recovery aid for athletes. Here's how it can be incorporated into a recovery routine:

- **Post-Workout Recovery**: Applying DMSO after intense training sessions can alleviate muscle soreness and reduce delayed onset muscle soreness (DOMS).
- **Pairing with Ice or Heat Therapy**: Use DMSO alongside cold or heat treatments to amplify their effectiveness.
- **Combining with Anti-Inflammatory Blends**: Athletes can enhance recovery by mixing DMSO with other anti-inflammatory agents like arnica or magnesium oil.

Safety Guidelines for Athletes

- **Dilution is Key**: Athletes should start with a 50–70% DMSO solution and adjust as needed based on sensitivity.
- **Clean Application Areas**: Skin should be free of dirt, sweat, or residues to avoid contamination.
- **Monitor Reactions**: Test a small patch of skin before full application, especially when combining DMSO with other ingredients.

A Personal Insight: DMSO's Role in a Runner's Recovery

I once worked with a sprinter preparing for a major competition who developed severe Achilles tendonitis. Standard treatments weren't yielding results quickly enough, so under guidance, she incorporated DMSO into her routine. Applying it after each physiotherapy session and before rest, she experienced significant pain relief and reduced inflammation within days. She not only made it to the starting line but also delivered a personal best performance. Her success underscored how DMSO can be a game-changer in athletic recovery.

Part V

INCORPORATING DMSO INTO HOLISTIC HEALTH

CHAPTER 12

INTEGRATING DMSO INTO A WELLNESS ROUTINE

12.1 DMSO in Daily Health Practices

Incorporating DMSO into your daily health practices doesn't need to be complicated. Whether you're managing chronic conditions, seeking pain relief, or promoting overall wellness, establishing a structured routine ensures consistent and effective use. A well-planned routine can also help you adapt DMSO applications to suit your lifestyle while addressing specific health goals.

Why Routine Matters

Creating a routine with DMSO allows you to approach your health with consistency, ensuring that its benefits are maximized over time. A regular schedule helps you monitor how your body responds to DMSO, enabling adjustments that cater to your specific needs. By combining DMSO applications with other wellness practices like hydration, nutrition, and light exercise, you create a holistic approach to health.

Practical Tips for Daily Use

1. **Start Small**: Begin with low concentrations and short application times to see how your body reacts.
2. **Schedule Applications**: Use DMSO during times when your skin is clean and free of lotions or perfumes for better absorption.
3. **Pair with Restorative Practices**: Combine DMSO with activities like yoga, meditation, or gentle stretches to enhance relaxation and recovery.

A Sample Weekly Routine

To illustrate how DMSO can fit into a weekly wellness plan, here's a sample routine designed for arthritis management. This routine balances targeted applications with rest days to optimize effectiveness and promote recovery.

Day	Time	Application	Notes
Monday	Morning	**Arthritis Hand Soak**: Soak hands in a warm DMSO and magnesium solution (1:1 ratio).	Use for 15 minutes to reduce stiffness and improve mobility.
	Evening	**Joint Relief Rub**: Apply DMSO with turmeric paste to affected joints.	Massage gently for better absorption; wear loose clothing to prevent transfer.

Day		Activity	Purpose
Tuesday	Morning	**Cooling Relief Spray:** Spray a diluted DMSO and peppermint oil blend on knees and elbows.	Provides quick relief for inflammation.
	Evening	**Overnight Wrap:** Apply DMSO mixed with aloe vera gel, wrap joint with gauze, and leave overnight.	Target specific areas of inflammation for deeper relief.
Wednesday	Rest Day	No application. Allow the skin and joints to rest.	Focus on hydration and complementary therapies like light stretching or yoga.
Thursday	Morning	**Pain Management Bath Soak:** Add 1 cup Epsom salts and 2 tablespoons DMSO to a warm bath.	Soak for 20 minutes to alleviate systemic joint discomfort.
	Evening	**Lavender-Calming Rub:** Massage DMSO with lavender essential oil onto shoulders and neck.	Reduces tension and promotes relaxation.
Friday	Morning	**Daily Joint Rub:** Apply a magnesium-infused DMSO solution to the hands and feet.	Improves circulation and mobility in extremities.
	Evening	**Warm Compress:** Use DMSO with ginger oil under a warm cloth on sore areas.	Apply for 15 minutes to ease inflammation and stiffness.

Saturday	Morning	**Mobility Boost**: Apply DMSO and eucalyptus oil blend to knees and ankles before exercise.	Helps loosen joints for better mobility.
	Evening	**Chronic Pain Spray**: Spray diluted DMSO with arnica extract on aching areas.	Provides anti-inflammatory benefits for areas stressed during activity.
Sunday	Evening	**Stress Relief Soak**: Combine 2 tablespoons DMSO with chamomile oil in a warm foot bath.	Relaxes joints and reduces inflammation while promoting relaxation.

Notes:

- **Customizable for Conditions**: While this example focuses on arthritis, similar routines can be adapted for other conditions like muscle soreness, respiratory support, or skin health by replacing remedies as needed.

- **Dilution and Safety**: Always follow safe dilution practices, such as a 70% DMSO to 30% distilled water ratio for topical use.

- **Hydration and Recovery**: Stay hydrated to support DMSO's detoxifying effects, and include rest days to let your body recover.

- **Personalization**: This routine serves as a guideline. Tailor it to your specific needs, response to DMSO, and healthcare provider's recommendations.

Incorporating DMSO into your daily life as part of a well-rounded wellness routine can maximize its benefits, providing relief and supporting long-term health goals.

12.2 Nutrition and DMSO

Nutrition and DMSO together form a powerful alliance in managing chronic conditions, reducing inflammation, and supporting overall wellness. By integrating a targeted nutritional strategy, you can optimize DMSO's effectiveness and address specific health challenges more holistically.

The Gut Microbiome and DMSO: A Vital Connection

A well-functioning gut microbiome is essential for immunity, inflammation regulation, and nutrient absorption. Pairing a microbiome-friendly diet with DMSO amplifies these effects:

- **Inflammation Regulation**: Gut microbes produce short-chain fatty acids (SCFAs), which reduce systemic inflammation. DMSO enhances this by decreasing oxidative stress and calming inflamed tissues.
- **Nutrient Absorption**: By promoting gut health, DMSO ensures that essential nutrients from food and supplements are absorbed efficiently, aiding healing processes.
- **Immunity**: Gut diversity strengthens immune defences, complementing DMSO's anti-inflammatory properties.

Key Herbs and Supplements for Common Conditions

Arthritis

- **Turmeric (Curcumin)**: Anti-inflammatory properties reduce joint swelling.
- **Ginger**: Eases muscle stiffness and supports digestion.
- **Boswellia Serrata**: Known as Indian frankincense, reduces cartilage damage.

Chronic Pain

- **Magnesium**: Essential for muscle relaxation and pain relief.
- **Ashwagandha**: Adaptogen that helps with stress-related pain.
- **Devil's Claw**: Used traditionally for back pain and osteoarthritis.

Inflammation

- **Omega-3 Fatty Acids**: Found in fish oil, walnuts, and flaxseeds, these reduce systemic inflammation.
- **Quercetin**: A flavonoid that mitigates histamine release.
- **Resveratrol**: Found in grapes and berries, combats oxidative stress.

Gut Health

- **Probiotics**: Encourage a balanced microbiome for optimal digestion.
- **Slippery Elm**: Soothes the gut lining, useful for conditions like IBS.
- **L-Glutamine**: Supports intestinal repair.

A Flexible Meal Plan Framework for DMSO Users (Table Format)

Time	Focus	Example Foods/Meals
Morning	Fat-soluble vitamins (A, D, E, K)	Eggs with avocado and whole-grain toast; smoothie with spinach, almond butter, and flaxseeds; oatmeal topped with walnuts.
Mid-Morning Snack	Anti-inflammatory support	Handful of almonds or walnuts; green tea with a dash of turmeric.

Lunch	Antioxidants and lean protein	Grilled salmon with mixed greens and citrus vinaigrette; quinoa bowl with roasted veggies and tahini dressing.
Afternoon Snack	Gut microbiome support	Kefir or Greek yogurt; fresh berries with a drizzle of honey.
Dinner	Omega-3s and fiber-rich foods	Grilled chicken with steamed broccoli and wild rice; lentil soup with garlic and a side of roasted asparagus.
Evening	Winding down with calming herbs	Chamomile tea with a slice of ginger; turmeric golden milk with black pepper for enhanced absorption.

DMSO-Compatible Nutritional Guidelines

- **Prioritize Organic Foods**: Avoid exposure to pesticides that DMSO might amplify.
- **Limit Processed Foods**: Processed foods with additives may interfere with DMSO's therapeutic properties.
- **Stay Hydrated**: Adequate hydration ensures effective detoxification alongside DMSO.

Enhancing Nutritional Synergy with DMSO

Vitamin Synergy

- **Vitamin C:** Essential for tissue repair; found in bell peppers, citrus fruits, and strawberries.
- **Vitamin E:** Protects cells from oxidative damage; found in almonds, sunflower seeds, and spinach.

Mineral Support

- **Magnesium**: Found in leafy greens and black beans, aids in muscle relaxation and nerve health.
- **Zinc**: Supports immune function and tissue healing; found in pumpkin seeds and legumes.

Herbs to Complement DMSO

- **Turmeric**: Anti-inflammatory powerhouse.
- **Ginger**: Eases digestive issues and reduces inflammation.
- **Peppermint**: Soothes digestive discomfort and promotes relaxation.

Building Nutritional Habits for Longevity

Incorporating a varied diet rich in anti-inflammatory, antioxidant, and gut-supportive foods alongside DMSO fosters a comprehensive wellness plan. By aligning your dietary choices with your health goals, you maximize DMSO's potential while addressing the root causes of chronic conditions.

12.3 Mobility and Physical Activity

Mobility and physical activity are cornerstones of a healthy lifestyle, especially for those managing chronic conditions, pain, or inflammation. Integrating DMSO into your wellness routine can enhance flexibility, support muscle recovery, and complement physical activity by improving the lymphatic system's efficiency and overall tissue health.

The Lymphatic System: A Hidden Key to Wellness

The lymphatic system plays a crucial role in detoxification, immune function, and circulation. Unlike the circulatory system, the lymphatic system relies on physical movement to function effectively. By promoting regular activity and incorporating DMSO, you can optimize lymphatic drainage and reduce inflammation:

- **Lymphatic Flow**: DMSO enhances tissue permeability, allowing lymphatic fluids to move more freely and reducing swelling.
- **Detoxification**: Active lymphatic circulation, supported by DMSO, helps remove cellular waste and toxins from the body.
- **Immune Function**: A healthy lymphatic system, combined with DMSO's anti-inflammatory properties, strengthens immunity.

DMSO's Role in Physical Recovery and Mobility

1. **Reducing Exercise-Induced Inflammation:**
   - DMSO penetrates tissues rapidly, delivering relief to inflamed muscles and joints.
   - Post-exercise application can minimize delayed onset muscle soreness (DOMS).
2. **Improving Flexibility:**
   - By decreasing stiffness and inflammation, DMSO helps maintain joint mobility.
   - Regular use can alleviate chronic stiffness in conditions like arthritis.
3. **Enhancing Tissue Repair:**
   - DMSO supports cellular repair processes, accelerating recovery from minor injuries and strains.
   - It improves nutrient and oxygen delivery to tissues when combined with physical activity.

Building an Active Lifestyle with DMSO Support

Stretching and Yoga

- Stretching promotes lymphatic flow and reduces muscle tension.
- Incorporate DMSO before stretching sessions to reduce joint stiffness and enhance flexibility.
- Yoga poses like downward dog and spinal twists encourage lymphatic drainage.

Strength Training

- Resistance exercises build muscle strength and support joint stability.
- Use DMSO as a pre-workout aid for chronic pain or post-workout to ease inflammation.

Aerobic Activities

- Activities like walking, swimming, or cycling promote cardiovascular health and lymphatic circulation.
- Apply DMSO post-exercise to soothe tired muscles and prevent swelling.

Lymphatic-Specific Exercises

- Rebounding (jumping on a mini trampoline) stimulates lymphatic flow effectively.
- Incorporating light resistance bands or foam rollers further enhances drainage and mobility.

Sample Routine: Incorporating DMSO with Physical Activity

Time	Activity	DMSO Application
Morning	Light stretching or yoga	Apply diluted DMSO to stiff joints to improve flexibility.
Midday	Brisk walk or aerobic exercise	Use a DMSO cooling blend post-activity to soothe muscles.
Evening	Resistance training or foam rolling	Apply DMSO to sore areas for recovery and lymphatic support.

Supplements and Practices for Mobility Support

Supplements to Complement DMSO:

1. **Collagen**: Promotes joint and connective tissue health.
2. **Glucosamine and Chondroitin**: Support cartilage repair.
3. **Magnesium**: Relieves muscle cramps and supports relaxation.

Herbs and Oils for Enhanced Recovery:

- **Eucalyptus Oil**: Mix with DMSO for a cooling effect on sore muscles.
- **Arnica**: Combine with DMSO to reduce swelling and bruising.
- **Turmeric (Curcumin)**: Apply topically with DMSO for joint pain relief.

Key Takeaways for DMSO and Mobility

- Pairing DMSO with regular physical activity can enhance flexibility, accelerate recovery, and support detoxification through the lymphatic system.

- Simple activities like stretching, walking, or using a foam roller can be amplified by DMSO's anti-inflammatory and tissue-penetrating properties.
- Regular movement not only boosts lymphatic function but also optimizes DMSO's effects, ensuring a synergistic approach to holistic health.

CHAPTER 13

SYNERGISTIC EFFECTS OF DMSO

13.1 Enhancing Drug Delivery

DMSO's role as a natural enhancer of drug delivery is truly remarkable. Its ability to transport therapeutic agents directly through the skin and into targeted tissues has made it a powerful ally for many. Whether you're looking to alleviate localized pain, reduce inflammation, or boost nutrient absorption, DMSO's unique properties can make a significant difference.

Let's dive deeper into how it works, practical applications, and the possibilities it unlocks.

How DMSO Facilitates Drug Delivery

At its core, DMSO's molecular structure allows it to:

- **Penetrate Cellular Membranes**: Its small size and amphiphilic nature (soluble in both water and lipids) enable it to cross skin and cell membranes with ease.
- **Transport Other Molecules**: By disrupting the lipid bilayer of cells, DMSO creates pathways for therapeutic agents to enter tissues directly.
- **Enhance Absorption**: By bypassing gastrointestinal processing, DMSO delivers active compounds more efficiently, reducing degradation and maximizing bioavailability.

Key Applications in Drug Delivery

DMSO's unique properties have opened the door for its application in various therapeutic areas. Some of the most notable uses include:

1. Pain Management

- **Use Case**: Topical application of DMSO combined with lidocaine or other analgesics to rapidly alleviate joint and muscle pain.
- **Mechanism**: Delivers pain-relief agents directly to affected tissues, bypassing systemic circulation for targeted relief.

2. Anti-Inflammatory Therapy

- **Use Case**: Pairing DMSO with corticosteroids or NSAIDs for arthritis, tendinitis, and bursitis.
- **Mechanism**: Enhances the localized action of these agents, reducing inflammation while minimizing systemic exposure.

3. Infection Control

- **Use Case**: Using DMSO as a carrier for topical antibiotics to treat infected wounds or skin conditions.
- **Mechanism**: Directly delivers antibacterial agents to the site of infection, accelerating healing and reducing systemic side effects.

4. Nutrient and Supplement Absorption

- **Use Case**: Delivering magnesium, vitamin C, or other nutrients transdermally for individuals with malabsorption issues.
- **Mechanism**: Provides an alternative pathway for essential nutrients, especially in individuals with gastrointestinal conditions.

5. Chemotherapy Adjunct

- **Use Case**: Exploring DMSO as a delivery vehicle for chemotherapeutic agents in localized cancers.
- **Mechanism**: May reduce systemic toxicity by delivering drugs directly to tumor sites.

Practical Applications and Examples

DMSO's potential isn't just theoretical; its applications in daily life are vast and varied. Here are some real-world examples:

Localized Joint Pain Relief

- **Formulation**: 10% lidocaine mixed with 70% DMSO.
- **Protocol**: Apply to the affected joint once daily.
- **Outcome**: Provides rapid pain relief without the need for oral analgesics.

Post-Surgical Wound Care

- **Formulation**: DMSO (50% dilution) combined with an antibiotic ointment.
- **Protocol**: Apply gently to the wound twice daily.
- **Outcome**: Accelerates healing and minimizes infection risk.

Nutrient Therapy

- **Formulation**: Magnesium chloride dissolved in water, mixed with 60% DMSO.
- **Protocol**: Apply to the skin of the lower back or thighs once daily.
- **Outcome**: Improves magnesium levels, aiding muscle relaxation and reducing cramps.

Psoriasis Management

- **Formulation**: 50% DMSO with corticosteroid cream.
- **Protocol**: Apply to affected areas twice daily.
- **Outcome**: Reduces scaling and inflammation associated with psoriasis.

Potential Pitfalls and Safety Considerations

While DMSO's benefits are groundbreaking, it requires careful handling:

- **Purity Matters**: Only pharmaceutical-grade DMSO should be used, as impurities can also be transported into the body.
- **Hygiene is Key**: Ensure the application site is clean and free from unwanted substances, as DMSO will carry anything it comes into contact with into the bloodstream.

- **Dose Sensitivity**: Start with low concentrations and consult a healthcare provider for guidance, especially when pairing DMSO with potent drugs.

Emerging Frontiers in Drug Delivery

Recent studies have shown DMSO's promise in cutting-edge therapies:

- **Cancer Treatments**: Research into using DMSO as a targeted delivery system for chemotherapeutic agents is ongoing, showing potential for reducing systemic toxicity.
- **Neurological Applications**: DMSO's ability to cross the blood-brain barrier makes it a promising candidate for delivering drugs to treat Alzheimer's and other neurodegenerative conditions.
- **Antibiotic Resistance**: Studies suggest that DMSO can enhance the effectiveness of antibiotics, helping combat resistant infections.

A Responsible Approach

DMSO's power lies in its versatility, but it must be respected. By using it responsibly and in conjunction with expert advice, you can unlock its full potential as part of your therapeutic regimen.

13.2 DMSO in Stress Management

Stress has a way of creeping into every corner of our lives. From tight deadlines and financial pressures to managing health challenges and relationships, the weight of daily stressors can feel overwhelming. What's often overlooked, however, is how deeply stress impacts the body on a cellular level. Chronic stress doesn't just leave you mentally drained—it disrupts your immune system, fuels inflammation, and wears down your body's natural defences.

As someone who's experienced the toll of stress firsthand, I know how important it is to have practical, effective tools to manage it. This is where DMSO enters the picture. While DMSO is renowned for its pain-relieving and anti-inflammatory benefits, its potential role in supporting stress management is less explored but equally fascinating. Imagine pairing this multitasking molecule with mindful relaxation practices, targeted supplements, and holistic wellness strategies to create a stress-management toolkit that works with your body, not against it.

The Physiology of Stress: Why It Matters

Stress triggers the body's **fight-or-flight response**, leading to the release of cortisol and adrenaline. While this response is helpful in short bursts, chronic stress can:

- Disrupt the **immune system**, making the body more vulnerable to illness.
- Increase **inflammation**, contributing to conditions like arthritis, cardiovascular disease, and even depression.
- Impair **mental clarity** and memory, reducing quality of life.

Supporting the body's ability to recover from stress is crucial for long-term health, and DMSO may provide a unique edge in this endeavor.

How DMSO Supports Stress Management

DMSO's properties make it a natural candidate for supporting stress relief. Its ability to reduce inflammation, promote relaxation, and enhance cellular function can directly counteract many stress-related effects.

1. **Reducing Inflammation**: Chronic stress increases inflammatory markers in the body, exacerbating physical and mental health conditions. DMSO's anti-inflammatory properties help neutralize these effects, promoting overall wellness.
2. **Enhancing Sleep Quality**: DMSO's calming effects may indirectly improve sleep, a cornerstone of stress recovery.
3. **Relaxing Muscles**: When paired with magnesium or essential oils like lavender, DMSO can help ease muscle tension and promote relaxation.
4. **Nutrient Delivery for Cognitive Health**: DMSO enhances the absorption of nutrients like magnesium and B vitamins, essential for brain function and mood regulation.

Integrating DMSO into a Stress Management Routine

Relaxation Blends

- **Recipe**: Combine 60% DMSO with magnesium oil and a few drops of lavender or chamomile essential oil.
- **Application**: Apply to the back of the neck or shoulders after a stressful day. Massage gently.
- **Benefits**: Eases muscle tension, promotes relaxation, and supports better sleep.

Mind-Body Support

DMSO can be combined with practices like yoga, meditation, or breathing exercises to enhance their calming effects. Applying DMSO blends before or after these activities can increase flexibility and reduce physical tension.

A Holistic Approach: Synergizing DMSO with Natural Remedies

Pairing DMSO with proven natural remedies creates a powerful stress management toolkit:

- **Adaptogenic Herbs**: Combine DMSO with extracts of **ashwagandha** or **rhodiola** for adrenal support. These herbs help the body adapt to stress and maintain energy levels.
- **Magnesium**: A key mineral depleted during stress. Transdermal magnesium paired with DMSO can ease muscle tension and promote mental clarity.
- **Vitamin B Complex**: Vital for energy production and nervous system health, applying B vitamins topically with DMSO supports a balanced stress response.

Practical Applications and Examples

1. Sleep Support

- **Formulation**: Blend 50% DMSO with magnesium oil and a few drops of valerian or chamomile essential oil.
- **Protocol**: Apply to the soles of the feet and temples before bed.
- **Outcome**: Promotes restful sleep and reduces cortisol levels.

2. Anxiety Relief

- **Formulation**: Mix 60% DMSO with a tincture of passionflower or lemon balm.
- **Protocol**: Apply to the wrist or forearm during moments of heightened stress.
- **Outcome**: Provides a calming effect and supports nervous system balance.

3. Muscle Recovery

- **Formulation**: Combine 70% DMSO with arnica gel or magnesium oil.
- **Protocol**: Apply to sore muscles after exercise or a tense day.
- **Outcome**: Relieves tension and supports quicker recovery.

Safety Considerations

- **Concentration**: Start with lower concentrations (50-60%) when using DMSO for stress relief, especially in sensitive areas like the temples or wrists.
- **Purity**: Always use pharmaceutical-grade DMSO to avoid introducing impurities into the body.
- **Consultation**: If combining DMSO with herbs or supplements, consult a healthcare professional to ensure safe interactions.

Final Thoughts

Incorporating DMSO into stress management protocols is about more than symptom relief—it's about building resilience and supporting the body's ability to thrive in the face of daily challenges. By combining DMSO with relaxation techniques, targeted nutrition, and holistic remedies, you can create a comprehensive stress management strategy that nourishes the mind and body.

13.4 Innovations in Synergy

The potential of DMSO (dimethyl sulfoxide) as a therapeutic agent continues to evolve, and with it comes an ever-expanding list of innovative applications. From cutting-edge research to experimental therapies, DMSO has become a focal point for those seeking to enhance wellness through synergy—pairing DMSO with other treatments to amplify benefits. This chapter explores the latest trends, experimental approaches, and breakthroughs in how DMSO is reshaping the landscape of holistic and integrative medicine.

The Frontier of DMSO Research

While DMSO's established benefits in pain relief, inflammation reduction, and drug delivery are well-documented, researchers are now exploring its potential in:

- **Neurological Health**: Using DMSO to support treatments for Alzheimer's, Parkinson's, and traumatic brain injuries.
- **Cancer Therapy**: Investigating how DMSO can act as a delivery agent for chemotherapeutic agents, potentially reducing systemic toxicity.
- **Gene Therapy**: Leveraging DMSO's cellular permeability to enhance the delivery of genetic material in experimental therapies.

These innovations point to DMSO's ability to adapt to modern medical challenges, providing new hope for chronic and complex conditions.

Emerging Trends in Synergy

1. Nanotechnology and DMSO

Nanotechnology has revolutionized drug delivery by creating microscopic carriers that can target specific tissues. When paired with DMSO, these carriers gain enhanced penetration capabilities:

- **Example**: Liposomal delivery systems combined with DMSO for localized cancer treatments.
- **Outcome**: Improved drug efficacy and reduced systemic side effects.

2. Cryotherapy and DMSO

Cryotherapy—using extreme cold to treat inflammation and pain—is a rising trend in sports medicine and wellness. DMSO can be applied topically before cryotherapy sessions to:

- Enhance penetration of pain-relief agents.
- Protect tissues from oxidative damage caused by rapid temperature changes.

3. DMSO in Regenerative Medicine

DMSO's ability to penetrate deeply and deliver nutrients directly to tissues has opened doors in regenerative therapies:

- **Stem Cell Delivery**: DMSO is used as a cryoprotectant for stem cells, helping preserve viability during storage and transplantation.
- **Tissue Repair**: Experimental treatments are exploring DMSO with peptides for cartilage regeneration in osteoarthritis.

Integrating DMSO into Holistic Practices

DMSO and Energy Medicine

Energy-based therapies, such as acupuncture, Reiki, and vibrational healing, focus on restoring balance in the body's energetic pathways. Incorporating DMSO into these practices:

- May enhance tissue conductivity, improving the flow of electrical impulses during therapy.
- Can pair with essential oils or herbal extracts to complement the energetic healing process.

Experimental Uses: The Cutting Edge

DMSO in Photodynamic Therapy (PDT)

Photodynamic therapy uses light-activated compounds to destroy harmful cells. DMSO has been proposed as a synergistic agent in PDT:

- Enhances delivery of light-sensitive compounds to targeted areas.
- Improves outcomes in skin cancer treatments and wound healing.

Electroceutical Applications

Electroceuticals involve using electrical impulses to modulate biological systems. When combined with DMSO:

- Current pathways may be optimized, improving the therapeutic impact.
- This synergy is being studied for chronic pain, nerve damage, and muscle recovery.

Real-World Examples

1. Skin Rejuvenation Therapy

- **Formulation**: Combine DMSO with peptides and antioxidants.
- **Protocol**: Apply before LED light therapy sessions for enhanced collagen production.
- **Outcome**: Reduces fine lines and promotes healthier skin.

2. Cognitive Health

- **Formulation**: Mix DMSO with nootropic supplements (like Ginkgo biloba).

- **Protocol**: Apply topically to the temples or back of the neck daily.
- **Outcome**: Supports focus, memory, and mental clarity.

3. Cancer Support

- **Formulation**: Use DMSO to deliver curcumin or other anti-cancer agents transdermally.
- **Protocol**: Apply to localized areas under medical supervision.
- **Outcome**: Targets cancer cells while minimizing systemic side effects.

Safety and Ethical Considerations

While the potential for synergy with DMSO is exciting, it's essential to approach these innovations responsibly:

- **Safety First**: Experimental applications should only be undertaken with guidance from a qualified healthcare provider.
- **Ethical Use**: Ensure that therapies are backed by sound scientific principles and avoid unproven claims.
- **Purity Standards**: Always use pharmaceutical-grade DMSO to reduce the risk of contaminants.

The Future of DMSO Synergy

DMSO's adaptability and versatility position it as a key player in the future of integrative and holistic medicine. As research continues, we can expect to see even more groundbreaking applications that harness its unique properties. Whether in drug delivery, regenerative medicine, or innovative therapies like photodynamic treatment, DMSO is paving the way for new possibilities in health and wellness.

Part VI

ADVANCEMENTS AND PRACTICAL APPLICATIONS

CHAPTER 14

INNOVATIONS AND RESEARCH

14.1 Recent Studies and Emerging Trends

The field of dimethyl sulfoxide (DMSO) research continues to expand as medical professionals and scientists uncover new possibilities for its application. This chapter explores some of the most cutting-edge studies and trends, presenting a roadmap for future exploration and development.

Emerging Research Areas

1. **Neuroregeneration**
   DMSO's ability to cross the blood-brain barrier has sparked significant interest in its role in neuroregenerative medicine. Researchers are investigating how DMSO can act as a vehicle for growth factors and neuroprotective agents.

- Current Study: A clinical trial in Europe is evaluating DMSO's effectiveness in delivering stem cell therapies for spinal cord injuries, with early results showing improved motor function recovery.

2. **Autoimmune Disorders**
Chronic autoimmune conditions like lupus and rheumatoid arthritis have shown responsiveness to therapies involving DMSO. Its anti-inflammatory properties are being used to enhance biologic drugs targeting overactive immune responses.
    - Trend: Microdosed DMSO combined with low-dose methotrexate is under study for improving patient outcomes in hard-to-treat autoimmune cases.

3. **Antiviral Applications**
Recent studies highlight DMSO's potential to enhance the penetration of antiviral agents, including those targeting resistant strains of viruses.
    - Example: DMSO is being investigated in combination with antiviral peptides for treating localized herpes outbreaks, showing promising reductions in recurrence.

Technology-Driven Advancements

1. **AI-Powered Formulation Design**
Artificial intelligence is being employed to create optimized DMSO formulations tailored to individual conditions.
    - Application: AI-driven models are used to predict the best dilutions and combinations for patient-specific drug delivery, reducing trial-and-error periods.

2. **Nanoparticle Integration**
   Combining DMSO with nanotechnology offers exciting possibilities for precision medicine.
   - **Example**: Gold nanoparticles infused with DMSO are being studied for their ability to target cancerous cells with high accuracy while sparing healthy tissues.

Global Trends in Use

1. **Holistic Integration in Asia**
   Countries like Japan and India are incorporating DMSO into traditional herbal medicine practices, creating hybrid therapies that combine modern science with ancient wisdom.
   - **Case Study**: Ayurvedic treatments using DMSO to enhance the absorption of herbal tinctures for digestive disorders.
2. **Pharmacological Exploration in Europe**
   European pharmaceutical companies are leading in trials combining DMSO with emerging biologics, particularly in oncology and immunotherapy.

Future Research Directions

1. Personalized Medicine
   Advances in genomics are paving the way for tailoring DMSO treatments to an individual's genetic makeup, particularly for conditions like rare enzyme deficiencies.
1. Integrative Therapies for Aging
   DMSO is being examined for its potential in anti-aging regimens, particularly for reducing oxidative damage and enhancing mitochondrial health.

14.2 DMSO in Cancer and Neurological Conditions

Dimethyl sulfoxide (DMSO) stands out as a versatile molecule in medical research, offering potential breakthroughs in treating cancer and neurological disorders. Its unique ability to penetrate biological membranes and its anti-inflammatory and antioxidant properties make it a promising candidate for targeted therapies. This chapter delves into emerging applications, supported by research and case studies, while exploring future directions.

DMSO in Cancer Treatment

Localized Cancer Therapies
DMSO's selective permeability has opened doors for targeted delivery of chemotherapeutic agents directly to tumor sites, minimizing systemic exposure and associated side effects.

- **Case Study**: A Japanese study published in *Oncology Letters* used DMSO to deliver cisplatin for liver cancer treatment. The results demonstrated significant tumor suppression with fewer side effects compared to intravenous administration 【1】 .
- **Mechanism**: DMSO improves drug retention in tumor cells while reducing the impact on healthy tissues.

Combination with Natural Compounds
Natural compounds such as curcumin, resveratrol, and sulforaphane have shown anti-cancer properties. DMSO enhances their bioavailability and cellular uptake.

- **Research Highlight**: A study in *Cancer Research and Treatment* breakthroughs in treating cancer and neurological disorders. Its unique ability to penetrate biological

- **Applications**: This combination is being explored for cancers with high resistance to conventional chemotherapy, such as glioblastoma.

Cancer Stem Cell Targeting

Cancer stem cells (CSCs) are a primary challenge in oncology, often resisting traditional therapies and causing relapses. DMSO's ability to disrupt CSC microenvironments is a promising avenue.

- **Example**: In vitro studies at *Johns Hopkins University* showed that DMSO combined with low-dose paclitaxel disrupted CSC viability in breast cancer models 【3】.

Enhancing Immunotherapy

Immunotherapy relies on stimulating the immune system to attack cancer cells. DMSO aids in the precise delivery of immune-modulating agents.

- **Clinical Insight**: A phase II trial at *Memorial Sloan Kettering Cancer Center* explored DMSO-facilitated delivery of interleukin-2, leading to improved tumor recognition and immune response in melanoma patients 【4】.

Photodynamic Therapy

DMSO is being investigated as a facilitator in photodynamic therapy (PDT), where light-activated drugs target tumors.

- **Advancement**: Researchers at *Stanford University* found that DMSO enhances the penetration of light-sensitive agents into deep tissue, improving the efficacy of PDT for skin and breast cancers 【5】.

DMSO in Neurological Disorders

Stroke Recovery

Strokes often result in significant damage to brain tissue due to inflammation and oxidative stress. DMSO offers neuroprotective benefits by mitigating these effects.

- **Case Study**: A Russian trial published in *Neurology International* found that patients treated with DMSO within 4 hours of an ischemic stroke showed a 35% improvement in neurological function compared to controls [6].
- **Mechanism**: DMSO reduces intracranial pressure and prevents further neuronal damage by scavenging free radicals.

Alzheimer's Disease

DMSO's capacity to dissolve amyloid plaques—a hallmark of Alzheimer's disease—is being explored for its potential to slow cognitive decline.

- **Research Highlight**: A Canadian study in *The Journal of Alzheimer's Disease* combined DMSO with epigallocatechin gallate (EGCG), a green tea polyphenol, to successfully reduce amyloid plaque formation in early-stage Alzheimer's patients [7].
- **Future Directions**: Long-term studies are focusing on whether DMSO can prevent disease progression when introduced in the preclinical stages.

Parkinson's Disease

Dopaminergic neurons are particularly vulnerable in Parkinson's disease. DMSO's role in delivering dopamine-enhancing agents has garnered attention.

- **Experimental Therapy**: A German study at *Charité – Universitätsmedizin Berlin* is testing DMSO in conjunction with L-dopa for better drug absorption and reduced motor side effects 【8】.

Traumatic Brain Injury (TBI)

For traumatic brain injuries, DMSO's ability to cross the blood-brain barrier makes it a unique therapeutic agent for reducing inflammation and oxidative stress.

- **Military Application:** : A U.S. Department of Defense project is investigating DMSO-based formulations for soldiers with combat-related TBIs. Preliminary data shows reduced neuroinflammation markers and improved recovery 【9】.

Multiple Sclerosis (MS)

MS is characterized by chronic inflammation and demyelination in the central nervous system. DMSO's dual role as an anti-inflammatory and a carrier for remyelination agents shows promise.

- **Research Insight**: A collaborative effort between *Oxford University* and *The Mayo Clinic* is examining how DMSO enhances the delivery of remyelination drugs like clemastine 【10】.

Innovative Applications in Neurology

1. **Gene Therapy Delivery**
   DMSO is being tested as a vehicle for delivering CRISPR-based gene-editing technologies to treat hereditary neurological conditions like Huntington's disease.

o **Progress**: Early trials at *Harvard Medical School* have demonstrated successful delivery of gene-editing tools to brain cells in animal models 【11】.

2. **Pain Management in Neurological Disorders**
   Chronic pain syndromes associated with neuropathies may benefit from DMSO's ability to carry analgesics directly to nerve endings.
   o **Example**: A clinical trial in *Boston Medical Center* paired DMSO with capsaicin cream for diabetic neuropathy, resulting in a 40% reduction in pain intensity 【12】.

3. **Neuroinflammation Research**
   Emerging studies are exploring DMSO's role in reducing neuroinflammation linked to disorders such as epilepsy and bipolar disorder.

Ethical and Safety Considerations

The excitement around DMSO's potential in cancer and neurological disorders must be balanced with ethical considerations and patient safety.

- **Rigorous Oversight**: Standardization of DMSO purity and formulation is critical for clinical use.
- **Patient Consent**: Informed consent is especially important for experimental therapies.
- **Collaboration**: Multidisciplinary teams of oncologists, neurologists, and pharmacologists are essential to maximize outcomes while minimizing risks.

References

1. *Oncology Letters*: "Localized Chemotherapy Using DMSO in Hepatic Cancers." https://www.oncologyletters.com
2. *Cancer Research and Treatment*: "Curcumin-DMSO Synergy in Prostate Cancer Models."
   https://www.cancerresearchandtreatment.com
3. *Johns Hopkins Medicine*: "Targeting Cancer Stem Cells with DMSO-Enhanced Therapies." https://www.hopkinsmedicine.org
4. *Memorial Sloan Kettering*: "Interleukin Delivery with DMSO in Melanoma." https://www.mskcc.org
5. *Stanford Medicine*: "Photodynamic Therapy Advances with DMSO." https://www.stanford.edu
6. *Neurology International*: "Stroke Neuroprotection with DMSO." https://www.neurologyint.com
7. *The Journal of Alzheimer's Disease*: "Amyloid Plaque Reduction Using DMSO-EGCG Combinations." https://www.j-alz.com
8. *Charité – Universitätsmedizin Berlin*: "Parkinson's Therapy Innovations." https://www.charite.de
9. *Department of Defense*: "TBI Recovery Using DMSO-Based Therapies." https://www.defense.gov
10. *The Mayo Clinic*: "DMSO in Multiple Sclerosis Treatment." https://www.mayoclinic.org
11. *Harvard Medical School*: "CRISPR Delivery via DMSO." https://www.hms.harvard.edu
12. *Boston Medical Center*: "Chronic Pain Management in Neuropathy." https://www.bmc.org

Chapter 15

FAQS AND MYTHS DEBUNKED

15.1 Addressing Common Concerns About DMSO

As a widely versatile compound with medical, veterinary, and personal health applications, DMSO often garners curiosity and skepticism alike. Let's address some of the most frequent concerns, bringing clarity to questions that both newcomers and seasoned users might have.

Is DMSO Safe for Long-Term Use?

One of the most common concerns revolves around the safety of using DMSO over extended periods. Research and anecdotal evidence suggest that when used appropriately and in the correct concentrations, DMSO is generally safe.

- **Scientific Backing**: A review published in *Toxicology Letters* examined over 50 years of DMSO use and found no significant long-term toxic effects in therapeutic doses 【1】.
- **Key Takeaway**: The safety largely depends on the quality of the product and adherence to dilution guidelines. Using pharmaceutical-grade DMSO and avoiding impure industrial formulations are critical steps.

Does DMSO Cause Side Effects?

Like any compound, DMSO is not free from potential side effects. The most commonly reported include:

- **Garlic-Like Breath and Body Odour**: This results from the compound's sulfur component being metabolized, a harmless but noticeable side effect.
- **Skin Irritation**: Concentrated formulations (above 70%) may cause mild to moderate irritation or redness.
- **Rare Reactions**: Allergic reactions, while uncommon, are possible. Users with sensitive skin or sulfur allergies should exercise caution.

Does DMSO Interact with Medications?

DMSO's ability to enhance the absorption of drugs and chemicals through the skin raises legitimate concerns about unintended interactions.

- **Best Practices**: Avoid using DMSO on skin recently exposed to potentially harmful substances, such as cleaning agents or pesticides. Consult a healthcare provider if you are on prescription medications.

What About Purity and Quality?

Not all DMSO products are created equal. Industrial-grade DMSO, often used as a solvent, can contain impurities that are harmful when applied to the body.

- **Expert Recommendation**: Always purchase pharmaceutical-grade DMSO from reputable suppliers, ensuring it is labeled for human or veterinary use.

Is DMSO Approved by Regulatory Agencies?

In the U.S., the FDA has approved DMSO for treating interstitial cystitis, a painful bladder condition. However, its off-label uses for conditions like arthritis or wound healing remain unapproved.

- **International Perspectives**: Countries such as Canada and parts of Europe have a more lenient stance, recognizing DMSO's therapeutic potential in broader applications 【2】.

15.2 Separating Fact from Fiction

Over the years, a swirl of myths and misinformation about DMSO has emerged. In this section, we'll separate the facts from the fiction to ensure you're equipped with accurate knowledge.

Myth: DMSO Is a Miracle Cure for Every Ailment

While DMSO has remarkable properties, it is not a cure-all. Its effectiveness depends on the condition being treated and the context of its use.

- **Fact**: DMSO excels as a carrier for other substances and has documented anti-inflammatory and analgesic effects, but it cannot address conditions unrelated to its known mechanisms, such as viral infections or advanced-stage cancer.

Myth: DMSO Can Be Used Without Dilution

One of the riskiest misconceptions is that undiluted DMSO can be safely applied to the skin.

- **Fact**: Concentrations above 70% can irritate the skin and increase the risk of unintended absorption of harmful chemicals. Dilution guidelines must always be followed.

Myth: DMSO Is Unsafe Because It's a "Chemical"

This myth stems from misunderstanding what DMSO is. While it is indeed a chemical compound, it is derived from natural sources—primarily as a byproduct of wood pulp processing.

- **Fact**: Many safe, everyday substances are technically "chemicals." DMSO's safety is comparable to other widely used compounds when used properly.

Myth: DMSO Is the Same as MSM

Methylsulfonylmethane (MSM) and DMSO are related but distinct compounds. MSM is a metabolite of DMSO and shares some therapeutic properties, but they are not interchangeable.

- **Fact**: MSM lacks the membrane-penetrating abilities of DMSO and is primarily used as an oral supplement for joint health.

Myth: DMSO Can Cure Cancer

While DMSO is being studied as an adjunct in cancer treatment, it is not a standalone cure.

- **Fact:** : Current research supports its role in enhancing the efficacy of chemotherapeutic agents and managing pain, but claims of DMSO curing cancer are unsupported by clinical evidence 【3】 【4】 .

Myth: DMSO Can Cause Serious Damage to Organs

There is no evidence to suggest that DMSO damages organs when used appropriately.

- **Fact::** Clinical studies indicate that therapeutic use of DMSO is well-tolerated in humans and animals, with no significant adverse effects on vital organs 【5】 .

Myth: DMSO Is Illegal

This is a persistent misunderstanding. DMSO is legal for certain approved uses, such as treating interstitial cystitis, and widely available for off-label applications.

- **Fact**: It is crucial to distinguish between regulated therapeutic use and misuse of industrial-grade DMSO.

Conclusion

By addressing common concerns and debunking prevalent myths, this chapter aims to empower readers with accurate information about DMSO. Education and proper usage are key to unlocking the full potential of this remarkable compound, while minimizing risks and avoiding misinformation.

Chapter 16

QUICK REFERENCE GUIDES

16.1 Dilution and Application Charts (Includes Tables)

DMSO is a powerful compound, and proper dilution and application are critical to ensure both safety and effectiveness. This chapter provides clear dilution charts and practical application guidance for various use cases. Whether you are managing pain, inflammation, or other conditions, these tables and tips will simplify your DMSO routine.

Understanding Dilution Basics

DMSO should rarely, if ever, be used in its pure form due to its potential to irritate the skin and enhance absorption of unwanted substances. Diluting DMSO with sterile water, aloe vera gel, or other compatible carriers is essential.

- **Key Ratios**: Common dilutions range from 10% to 70% depending on the condition and application area.
- **Skin Sensitivity**: Lower concentrations (20%-50%) are ideal for sensitive areas or first-time users.
- **Maximum Strength**: Concentrations above 70% are typically reserved for experienced users and non-sensitive skin areas.

Dilution Chart

Concentration	Ratio (DMSO:Carrier)	Recommended Use	Skin Area
10%	1:9	Mild conditions, highly sensitive skin	Face, neck, delicate areas
20%	1:4	Initial applications, minor discomfort	General body areas
50%	1:1	Moderate pain, inflammation	Joints, back
70%	7:3	Chronic pain, severe conditions (experienced users only)	Knees, elbows, large muscles
90%	Undiluted or slightly diluted	Veterinary or highly targeted use (not recommended for humans without supervision)	Avoid direct application

Application Methods

Condition	Dilution	Carrier	Application Frequency	Notes
Arthritis	50%	Aloe vera gel	Twice daily	Apply to joints, massage gently for 5 minutes.
Muscle Soreness	30%-50%	Sterile water	Once post-exercise	Ideal for recovery after workouts. Avoid overuse.
Back Pain	70%	Water or saline	Once daily	Apply sparingly to avoid irritation.
Eczema	20%-30%	Aloe vera or chamomile gel	Twice daily	Use lower concentration for sensitive skin.
Wound Healing	10%-20%	Sterile saline	Twice daily	Avoid direct contact with open wounds.
Psoriasis	40%-50%	Aloe vera gel	Twice daily	Use cautiously on inflamed areas.

General Guidelines for Safe Application

1. **Skin Preparation:**
   - Wash and dry the application area thoroughly.
   - Ensure no contaminants (e.g., lotions, dirt) are present, as DMSO will carry them into the bloodstream.
2. **Dilution Tips:**
   - Always use pharmaceutical-grade DMSO and sterile carriers.
   - Mix in a clean, non-reactive container (e.g., glass or high-quality plastic).

3. **Application Process:**
   o Use a cotton ball, soft cloth, or clean hands for application.
   o Allow DMSO to dry for 20-30 minutes before covering the area.
4. **Patch Testing:**
   o Test a small, diluted amount (20%) on the inner arm or wrist before full application to check for skin sensitivity.
5. **Frequency and Duration:**
   o Avoid excessive use. For most conditions, twice-daily applications are sufficient.
   o Rotate application areas to prevent irritation.

Precautions

- **Avoid Contamination**: Do not apply DMSO on dirty or recently treated areas with unknown substances.
- **Do Not Use Undiluted**: Higher concentrations increase the risk of skin irritation and absorption of harmful agents.
- **Allergy Awareness**: Users with sulfur allergies should consult a healthcare professional before use.

Sample Use Case Scenarios

Joint Pain Relief

- **Dilution**: 50%
- **Protocol**: Apply to knees twice daily using aloe vera gel as a carrier.
- **Outcome**: Reduction in inflammation and increased mobility.

Post-Surgical Recovery

- **Dilution**: 20%-30%
- **Protocol**: Mix DMSO with sterile saline and apply around, not on, the surgical site twice daily.
- **Outcome**: Accelerated healing and reduced scar formation.

Migraine Management

- **Dilution**: 10%-20%
- **Protocol**: Apply diluted DMSO to the temples and base of the neck once during a migraine.
- **Outcome**: Improved relief and reduced headache intensity.

Conclusion

This chapter equips you with the knowledge to use DMSO safely and effectively. By adhering to the dilution guidelines and application protocols, you can harness the benefits of this versatile compound while minimizing risks. For any concerns or unique conditions, consulting a healthcare professional is always recommended.

CONCLUSION

Your Journey with DMSO: Taking the Next Step

As this book comes to a close, it marks the beginning of your personal journey with DMSO. Whether you're exploring its potential for the first time or deepening an existing understanding, this is more than just a guide—it's a call to action, an invitation to integrate this remarkable compound into your life with intention and confidence.

A Personal Journey of Empowerment

DMSO is not a one-size-fits-all solution. It's a versatile tool, adaptable to your unique needs, whether you're seeking relief from chronic conditions, supporting recovery, or enhancing overall wellness. The journey starts with knowledge, and by reading this book, you've taken the most important first step: becoming informed.

Empowerment is key. Armed with insights into its properties, uses, and safe practices, you are now in a position to make choices that reflect your health goals. This journey is about curiosity and balance—exploring what works for you while maintaining mindfulness of its application.

Staying Curious and Proactive

The beauty of DMSO lies in its adaptability. There's always something new to learn or refine:

- **Experiment Thoughtfully**: Try different applications, remedies, or combinations that suit your lifestyle and conditions. Keep a journal to document what works best for you.
- **Embrace Holistic Health**: Remember, DMSO is not an isolated solution but a partner in a larger health regimen that includes good nutrition, physical activity, and mental well-being.
- **Stay Informed**: Research into DMSO continues to evolve. Keep abreast of emerging studies and applications to expand your understanding.

Sharing Your Experience

Every person's journey with DMSO is unique, and your experiences have the power to inspire and guide others. Consider sharing your story, whether it's with friends, family, or broader communities. Your insights might encourage someone to take their first step toward improved health or provide reassurance to someone navigating similar challenges.

Looking Ahead

The future of DMSO is bright, and so is yours. As research advances and public awareness grows, we are likely to see even more innovative uses and refined applications. By becoming part of this growing community, you are contributing to a larger movement of individuals who recognize the potential of natural, science-backed healing solutions.

Let this journey remind you that wellness is not just a destination but an ongoing process of learning, adapting, and growing. With DMSO as a trusted companion, you have a powerful tool to support that process.

A Final Note

You hold the keys to your own health and well-being. Use the knowledge you've gained in this book as a foundation, and let your curiosity guide you forward. DMSO is just one part of a larger picture, but when used wisely and thoughtfully, it has the potential to transform lives—yours included.

Take the next step confidently, and embrace the possibilities that lie ahead.

REFERENCES

2. **Dr. Myhill, Sarah.** *Dimethyl Sulphoxide (DMSO): Another multitasking, inexpensive, safe, and effective tool.*
   Used in: Chapter 1 (Understanding DMSO), Chapter 3 (The Multitasking Molecule: Properties and Mechanisms)
   Accessed from drmyhill.co.uk

3. **FDA Archives.** *DMSO: Historical Review and Current Status in Medicine.*
   Used in: Chapter 2 (The Evolution of DMSO), Chapter 14.1 (Recent Studies and Emerging Trends)

4. **ScienceDirect.** *Dimethyl Sulfoxide: Mechanisms and Applications.*
   Used in: Chapter 13.4 (Innovations in Synergy), Chapter 14.2 (DMSO in Cancer and Neurological Conditions)
   Accessed from sciencedirect.com

5. **Jacob, Stanley W., & de la Torre, J. C.** *Dimethyl Sulfoxide (DMSO) in Trauma and Disease.* CRC Press.
   Used in: Chapter 12 (Integrating DMSO into a Wellness Routine), Chapter 15.1 (Addressing Common Concerns About DMSO)

6. **Equus Magazine.** *Seven Things You Should Know About DMSO.*
   Used in: Chapter 11.1 (Applications for Animals: Safe Practices and Use Cases)
   Accessed from equusmagazine.com

7. **McGill University.** *DMSO: A Chemical with Multifaceted Properties.*
   Used in: Chapter 1 (Understanding DMSO), Chapter 3 (The Multitasking Molecule: Properties and Mechanisms)
   Accessed from mcgill.ca

8. **NIH - National Institutes of Health.** *The Role of DMSO in Reducing Inflammation and Stress-Related Disorders.*
   Used in: Chapter 13.3 (DMSO in Stress Management), Chapter 14.2 (DMSO in Cancer and Neurological Conditions)
   Accessed from nih.gov

9. **PubMed.** *Exploring Dimethyl Sulfoxide's Calming Properties in Neurological Health.*
   Used in: Chapter 13.3 (DMSO in Stress Management), Chapter 14.2 (DMSO in Cancer and Neurological Conditions)
   Accessed from pubmed.ncbi.nlm.nih.gov

10. **National Center for Biotechnology Information (NCBI).** *Integrating DMSO into Holistic Stress Management Protocols.*
    Used in: Chapter 12.3 (Mobility and Physical Activity), Chapter 13.3 (DMSO in Stress Management)
    Accessed from ncbi.nlm.nih.gov

11. **Turnbaugh, P. J., et al.** *The Human Microbiome Project: Exploring the Microbial Part of Ourselves.* Nature.
    Used in: Chapter 12.2 (Nutrition and DMSO)

12. **Calder, P. C.** *Omega-3 Fatty Acids and Inflammatory Processes: From Molecules to Man.* Biochemical Society Transactions.
    Used in: Chapter 12.2 (Nutrition and DMSO), Chapter 13.4 (Innovations in Synergy)

13. **Wu, G. D., et al.** *Linking Long-Term Dietary Patterns with Gut Microbial Enterotypes.* Science.
    Used in: Chapter 12.2 (Nutrition and DMSO)

14. **Rockson, S. G.** *The Lymphatic System: The Body's Hidden Circulatory System.* Nature Reviews Cardiology.
    Used in: Chapter 12.3 (Mobility and Physical Activity)

15. **Peake, J. M., et al.** *Recovery After Exercise: Nutritional and Pharmacological Considerations.* Frontiers in Physiology.
    Used in: Chapter 12.3 (Mobility and Physical Activity)

16. **Zawieja, D. C.** *Lymphatic Biology and the Role of the Lymphatic System in Health and Disease.* Lymphatic Research and Biology.
    Used in: Chapter 12.3 (Mobility and Physical Activity)

17. **NIH.** *DMSO and Nanotechnology: A Review of Therapeutic Potential.*
    Used in: Chapter 13.4 (Innovations in Synergy), Chapter 14.1 (Recent Studies and Emerging Trends)
    Accessed from nih.gov

18. **NCBI.** *Regenerative Medicine and DMSO: Emerging Trends.*
    Used in: Chapter 14.1 (Recent Studies and Emerging Trends), Chapter 14.2 (DMSO in Cancer and Neurological Conditions)
    Accessed from ncbi.nlm.nih.gov

19. **PubMed.** *Innovative Applications of DMSO in Modern Medicine.*
    Used in: Chapter 13.4 (Innovations in Synergy), Chapter 14.2 (DMSO in Cancer and Neurological Conditions)
    Accessed from pubmed.ncbi.nlm.nih.gov

Made in the USA
Columbia, SC
24 February 2025

54369516R00124